"The concept of the glycemic index has been distorted and bastardized by popular writers and diet gurus. Here at last, is a book that explains what we know about the glycemic index and its importance in designing a diet for optimum health. Carbohydrates are not all bad. Read the good news about pasta and even—believe it or not—sugar!"
—ANDREW WEIL, M.D., University of Arizona College of Medicine, author of *Spontaneous Healing* and *8 Weeks to Optimum Health*

■

"Forget *Sugar Busters*. Forget *The Zone*. If you want the real scoop on how carbohydrates and sugar affect your body, read this book by the world's leading researchers on the subject. It's the authoritative, last word on choosing foods to control your blood sugar."
—JEAN CARPER, best-selling author of *Miracle Cures, Stop Aging Now!* and *Food: Your Miracle Medicine*

■

"Mounting evidence indicates that refined carbohydrates and high glycemic index foods are contributing to the escalating epidemics of obesity and type 2 diabetes worldwide. This dietary pattern also appears to increase the risk of heart disease and stroke. The skyrocketing proportion of calories from added sugars and refined carbohydrates in westernized diets portends a future acceleration of these trends. *The Glucose Revolution* challenges traditional doctrines about optimal nutrition and the role of carbohydrates in health and disease. Brand-Miller and colleagues are to be congratulated for an eminently lucid and important book that explains the science behind the glycemic index and provides tools and strategies for modifying diet to incorporate this knowledge. I strongly recommend the book to both health professionals and the general public who could use this state-of-the-art information to improve health and well-being."

—JOANN E. MANSON, M.D., Dr.P.H.,
Professor of Medicine, Harvard Medical School
and Co-Director of Women's Health, Division of
Preventive Medicine, Brigham and Women's Hospital

■

"Here is at last a book explaining the importance of taking into consideration the glycemic index of foods for overall health, athletic performance, and in reducing the risk of heart disease and diabetes. The book clearly explains that there are different kinds of carbohydrates that work in different ways and why a universal recommendation to "increase the carbohydrate content of your diet" is plainly simple and scientifically inaccurate. Everyone should put the glycemic index approach into practice."

—ARTEMIS P. SIMOPOULOS, M.D.,
senior author of *The Omega Diet* and
The Healing Diet and President, The Center for
Genetics, Nutrition and Health, Washington, D.C.

"Although the jury is still out on the utility of the glycemic index, many of the curious will benefit from a careful reading of this book, and some will find that the glycemic index is particularly helpful for them. Everyone can enjoy the recipes, some of which are to die for!"
—JOHANNA DWYER, D. Sc., R.D.,
editor of *Nutrition Today*

Praise for
The Glucose Revolution Life Plan

"Delicious! *The Glucose Revolution Life Plan* diet worked wonderfully for me. Certainly the best and most sensible diet that I've seen in years."
—RICHARD N. PODELL, M.D., M.P.H.,
Clinical Professor, Department of Family Medicine,
UMDNJ-Robert Wood Johnson Medical School

■

"Finally, a nutrition book I can recommend to athletes! Every other book on the market meant for athletes recommends the same tired high-carbohydrate diet that promotes low macronutrient levels and ultimately poor endurance. *The Glucose Revolution Life Plan* points out that humans are not adapted to such a diet. Eating as is proposed here is optimal for human athletes as it maintains health and contributes to peak performance."
—JOEL FRIEL,
coach of Olympic-caliber endurance athletes

The Glucose Revolution Pocket Guide to
CHILDREN WITH TYPE 1 DIABETES

OTHER *GLUCOSE REVOLUTION* TITLES

The Glucose Revolution: The Authoritative Guide to the Glycemic Index—The Groundbreaking Medical Discovery

The Glucose Revolution Life Plan

■

The Glucose Revolution Pocket Guide to the Top 100 Low Glycemic Foods

The Glucose Revolution Pocket Guide to Diabetes

The Glucose Revolution Pocket Guide to Losing Weight

The Glucose Revolution Pocket Guide to Sports Nutrition

The Glucose Revolution Pocket Guide to Sugar and Energy

The Glucose Revolution Pocket Guide to Your Heart

The Glucose Revolution Pocket Guide to the Glycemic Index and Healthy Kids

The GLUCOSE Revolution

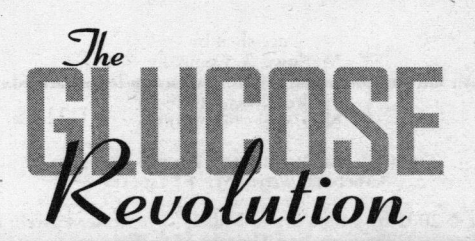

POCKET GUIDE TO

CHILDREN WITH TYPE 1 DIABETES

HEATHER GILBERTSON, B.S. GRAD. DIET.,
GRAD. CERT. DIAB. ED., APD

JENNIE BRAND-MILLER, PH.D.

KAYE FOSTER-POWELL, B.SC., M. NUTR. & DIET.

THOMAS M.S. WOLEVER, M.D., PH.D.

ADAPTED BY

JOHANNA BURANI, M.S., R.D., C.D.E.,
AND LINDA RAO, M.ED.

■

MARLOWE & COMPANY
NEW YORK

Published by
Marlowe & Company
An Imprint of Avalon Publishing Group Incorporated
841 Broadway, 4th Floor
New York, NY 10003

THE GLUCOSE REVOLUTION POCKET GUIDE TO
CHILDREN WITH TYPE 1 DIABETES

Copyright © 2001 by Jennie Brand-Miller, Kaye Foster-Powell, Heather Gilbertson, and Thomas M.S. Wolever

All rights reserved. No part of this book may be reproduced in whole or in part without written permission from the publisher, except by reviewers who may quote brief excerpts in connection with a review in a newspaper, magazine, or electronic publication; nor may any part of this book be reproduced, stored in a retrieval system, or transmitted in any form or by any means electronic, mechanical, photocopying, recording, or other, without written permission from the publisher.

Many factors can affect your child's blood sugar levels. If your child has diabetes and you are struggling to control her blood sugar, it's important to seek medical help. Your child's doctor may need to reassess how much she exercises, what she weighs and eats, her stress levels and her need for medication.

First published in Australia in 2001 under the title
The G.I. Factor The Glucose Revolution Pocket Guide for Children with Type 1 Diabetes by Hodder Headline Australia Pty Limited.

This edition is published by arrangement with
Hodder Headline Pty Limited

Library of Congress Cataloging-in-Publication Data

Brand-Miller, Janette, 1952-
  The glucose revolution pocket guide to children with type 1 diabetes / by Jennie Brand-Miller, Kaye Foster-Powell, and Thomas M.S. Wolever.
    p. cm.
  ISBN 1-56924-638-6
  1. Diabetes—Diet therapy. 2. Glycemic index I. Foster-Powell, Kay. II. Wolever, Thomas M.S. III. Title.

RC662 .B718 2001
616.4'620654—dc21

2001022218

9 8 7 6 5 4 3 2 1

Designed by Pauline Neuwirth, Neuwirth & Associates, Inc.

Printed in the United States of America
Distributed by Publishers Group West

CONTENTS

Preface ... xi
How to Use This Book ... xiii

PART 1:
THE GLUCOSE REVOLUTION AND DIABETES

1. What is the Glucose Revolution? ... 3
2. The Glycemic Index and Diabetes ... 5
3. Diabetes and Carbohydrates ... 8
4. What Type of Carbohydrate? ... 11
5. Sources of Carbohydrate ... 13
6. Why We Need More Carbohydrate ... 15
7. The Glycemic Index: Some Background ... 17
8. How We Measure the Glycemic Index ... 21

PART 2:
THE GLYCEMIC INDEX AND YOUR CHILD

9. Low G.I. Diets for Children ... 27
10. Who Benefits from Low G.I. Foods? ... 30
11. The Food Pyramid for Children ... 32
12. Blood Sugar and Exercise ... 34
13. Blood Sugar Guidelines ... 37
14. Handling Low Blood Sugar ... 39
15. Sick Day Hypoglycemia ... 43

PART 3:
FOOD BASICS

16. Cereals and Grain Foods ... 49
17. Vegetables ... 53
18. Fruit ... 55

19. Dairy Foods	57
20. Meat and Meat Alternatives	59
21. Fats and Oils	61
22. Sugar	63

PART 4:
AGE-SPECIFIC INFORMATION FOR DIABETIC CHILDREN

23. Babies	69
24. Toddlers and Pre-Schoolers	74
25. School-Age Children	78
26. Teenagers	82
27. The Food Pyramid for Adolescents and Teenagers	90

PART 5:
THE GLYCEMIC INDEX MENU PLANNER FOR CHILDREN AND TEENS

28. Breakfast	95
29. Lunches and Sandwich Fillers	99
30. Main Meals for Children and Teens	102
31. Just Desserts	106
32. Low G.I. Snacks	108
33. Party Ideas	110

PART 6:
YOUR QUESTIONS ANSWERED

The Meal Skippers	115
No Special Treats Required	117
Candy Concerns	118
Hypoglycemia After Sports	118
Infant and Toddler Concerns	119

PART 7:
THE G.I. TABLES

How to Use the G.I. Tables	125
The Glycemic Index Tables	127
For More Information	143
About the Authors	147
Acknowledgments	151

PREFACE

The Glucose Revolution and *The Glucose Revolution Life Plan* are the definitive, all-in-one guides to the glycemic index. To supplement that information, we've now written this pocket guide to show you how the glycemic index relates to children with type 1 diabetes. We'll describe how the glycemic index can reduce blood sugar levels and show you how easy it is to choose low G.I. foods that benefit your whole family.

In this volume, we offer more in-depth information about how the glycemic index affects children with diabetes than we had room to include in our other books: For example, we've included the questions that people most frequently ask about children's diabetes, nutrition and many other extras. For a more comprehensive discussion of the glycemic index and all its uses, please consult *The Glucose Revolution* and *The Glucose Revolution Life Plan*.

Please note: We have used the pronoun "she" throughout this book when describing a child with diabetes. We chose to use this word only in the interest of consistency, not to exclude boys or to imply in any way that girls are the only children affected by the disease.

HOW TO USE THIS BOOK

*M*any young people with diabetes, despite doing everything they are told, often find that their blood sugar levels remain too high. This pocket guide will help you to understand the glycemic index and how you can use it to help your child with type 1 diabetes. After eating the low G.I. way, your children will be well on the road to a lifetime of healthy eating that will help them to control their blood sugar and avoid diabetic complications. In this book, we:

- explain which types of carbohydrate are best for children with type 1 diabetes and why;
- how you how to include more of the right sort of carbohydrate in your children's diet;
- provide practical hints for meal preparation and tips to help make the glycemic index work throughout the day;
- give you lots of low G.I. menus that children (even picky eaters) will love; and
- include an A–Z listing of over 300 foods with their G.I. values, carbohydrate and fat grams.

■

THIS BOOK CONTAINS THE LATEST INFORMATION ABOUT CARBOHYDRATES AND THE OPTIMUM DIET FOR CHILDREN WITH DIABETES.

Part 1

THE GLUCOSE REVOLUTION AND DIABETES

WHAT IS THE GLUCOSE REVOLUTION?

THE GLYCEMIC INDEX AND DIABETES

DIABETES AND CARBOHYDRATES

WHAT TYPE OF CARBOHYDRATE?

SOURCES OF CARBOHYDRATE

WHY WE NEED MORE CARBOHYDRATE

THE GLYCEMIC INDEX: SOME BACKGROUND

HOW WE MEASURE THE GLYCEMIC INDEX

Chapter 1

WHAT IS THE GLUCOSE REVOLUTION?

In our first book, *The Glucose Revolution*, we explained that not all carbohydrates are created equal, and discussed how different types of carbohydrate work in different ways in our bodies. We revealed that some carbohydrates are absorbed much more slowly than others and that these slowly digested carbohydrates have startling health benefits for everybody. These carbohydrates:

- provide sustained energy;
- satisfy and reduce appetite;
- lower insulin levels, which makes you burn more—and store less—fat;
- help manage diabetes; and

- reduce diabetes, heart disease and certain cancer risks.

We also explained that eating the right *amount* of carbohydrate, as well as the right *type* of carbohydrate significantly contribute to our quality of life, health and well being.

The rate of carbohydrate digestion has important implications for everybody, but in this book we show how it can help young people with diabetes.

So whether you have type 1 diabetes yourself or care for someone who does, we believe that the G.I. value of carbohydrate foods is vital information that will help you with your day-to-day efforts at blood sugar control.

Our research has been described as a "glucose revolution" because it has turned many traditional beliefs about starchy foods upside down and has changed the way we think about carbohydrates forever!

■

THE GLUCOSE REVOLUTION CAN GIVE YOUNG PEOPLE WITH DIABETES A NEW LEASE ON LIFE!

■

Chapter 2

THE GLYCEMIC INDEX AND DIABETES

*N*ot long ago, people with diabetes were told to eat complex carbohydrates (starches) because it was believed these were slowly absorbed, causing a smaller rise in blood sugar levels. Doctors asked people with diabetes to restrict the amount of simple sugars they ate because these simple sugars were thought to be quickly absorbed, making blood sugar shoot up fast and high.

We now know that these assumptions were wrong. Different carbohydrate foods *do* have different effects on blood sugar levels, but we can't predict the effect by looking at the sugar or starch content. We know this because since the 1980s scientists have studied the actual blood sugar responses—of healthy people and people with diabetes—to hundreds of foods. Researchers asked people to eat everyday foods, then measured their blood sugar levels frequently for 2 or 3 hours after the meal.

To rank carbohydrates according to their true physiological effect on blood sugar levels, the scientists came up with the term "glycemic index." This is simply a ranking of foods from 0 to 100 that tells us whether a food will raise blood sugar levels dramatically, moderately or just a little.

The first surprise was that many starchy foods (bread, potatoes, crackers and many breakfast cereals) are digested and absorbed very quickly, not slowly as we had once assumed.

The next surprise was that moderate amounts of many sugary foods did not produce dramatic rises in blood sugar that we had thought. In fact, many foods containing sugar actually showed intermediate blood sugar responses, often lower than foods such as bread.

The glycemic index tells the true story: The old distinctions between starchy foods and sugary foods or simple versus complex carbohydrate have no scientific basis at all.

■

FORGET ABOUT SIMPLE AND COMPLEX CARBOHYDRATE, OR GOOD OR BAD FOODS. THINK GLUCOSE REVOLUTION!

■

WHY IS THE GLYCEMIC INDEX SO IMPORTANT IN DIABETES?

When a person has diabetes and her blood sugar isn't under control, it can cause damage to the blood vessels in the heart, legs, brain, eyes and kidneys. This is why heart attacks, strokes, kidney failure and blindness are more common in people with diabetes. High blood sugar levels can also damage the nerves in the feet, causing pain, irritation and numbness.

Low G.I. foods can help reduce the complications of diabetes by:

- improving blood sugar control, and
- improving blood fats.

Several studies show that a low G.I. diet lowers "bad" (LDL) cholesterol levels as it increases "good" (HDL) cholesterol. That's important because scientists think that increased levels of good HDL cholesterol protect against blood vessel disease and heart attack.

SLOWLY DIGESTED LOW G.I. FOODS HELP TO CONTROL BLOOD SUGAR LEVELS IN PEOPLE WITH DIABETES.

Chapter 3

DIABETES AND CARBOHYDRATES

*D*iabetes is a chronic condition in which the blood contains too much sugar. Normally, when we eat carbohydrate foods, our bodies break them down into a form that we can absorb and which our cells can use. This breaking-down process is digestion, the end product of which is blood glucose. (Digestion actually starts in the mouth as we chew our food and amylase, the digestive enzyme in saliva, is incorporated into the food.) Most digestion, however, takes place in the small intestine where enzymes break the large starch molecules down into simpler molecules. The resulting simple sugars (glucose, fructose and galactose) are absorbed from the small intestine into the bloodstream.

To keep blood sugar levels normal, we need the right amount of the hormone **insulin**. Insulin drives the sugar out of the blood and into the body's muscles, where it is used to provide energy for the body. If there isn't enough insulin or if the insulin doesn't do its job properly, we develop diabetes, of which there are two main types:

Type 1, or insulin-dependent, diabetes mellitus is most commonly diagnosed during childhood. In this type of diabetes, the pancreas doesn't produce enough insulin and a person needs multiple insulin injections every day to replace this insulin deficit. Since the amount of insulin injected is prescribed, it's important for the person to regulate food intake to maintain a balanced blood sugar level.

Although children and teenagers with type 1 diabetes are insulin-dependent, there are many steps they can take to reduce disease symptoms and complications. That's what this book is all about.

Type 2, or non insulin-dependent, diabetes mellitus usually occurs in people over 40, although the disease is now beginning to appear in younger people who are sedentary and overweight. People with type 2 diabetes can still make their own insulin, but either don't produce enough of it or produce insulin that doesn't work effectively. Exercise and eating a healthy diet is all that some people with type 2 diabetes have to do to keep their blood sugar levels within the normal range, while other people may need to take medication or insulin injections.

FOOD FOR THOUGHT

Carbohydrates include starchy foods such as bread, cookies, potatoes, breakfast cereals, pasta, rice and noodles, plus all the foods that contain natural or added sugar, such as fruit, milk, ice cream, jelly, chocolate, soft drinks and candy.

■

THE DIETARY GUIDELINES FOR CHILDREN WITH DIABETES ARE THE SAME AS THOSE FOR ALL CHILDREN AND TEENAGERS.

■

Chapter 4

WHAT TYPE OF CARBOHYDRATE?

Thanks to research on the glycemic index, we now know that even people with diabetes can enjoy foods containing added sugar (in moderation, of course) as part of a healthy diet. Sugar itself has only an intermediate G.I. value, which means that it has a moderate effect on blood sugar levels compared with other carbohydrate foods. In fact, many sugar-containing foods, such as yogurt and flavored milk, actually have low G.I. values and raise blood sugar levels less than some refined wheat products.

You may be familiar with the carbohydrate exchange system that for many years has helped people with diabetes determine how much carbohydrate they can eat. (It has also been used extensively in the past in some weight loss programs.) The glycemic index research, however, has scientifically proven that this system is flawed, because the exchange system assumes that equal amounts of different carbohydrate foods have similar effects on blood sugar levels. That's wrong. The change in blood sugar after one exchange of cornflakes, for example, is very different than after one exchange of apple.

Although the carbohydrate exchange system is a helpful guide to carbohydrate quantity, remember its limitations when it comes to predicting the impact of foods on your blood sugar levels.

FOUR TIPS FOR CHOOSING CARBOHYDRATES

- Use standard household measures such as ounces and cups to measure portions; the serving sizes listed on food labels aren't necessarily the amounts your child should eat.
- Your child should eat regular meals and snacks based on low G.I. carbohydrate foods.
- Choose your child's carbohydrate from a wide variety of sources—both starch and sugar foods.
- Use the G.I. tables to choose the most suitable carbohydrate for your child. Aim to include at least one low G.I. food in every meal and snack. (You'll find the G.I. Table on page 128.)

■

THE GLYCEMIC INDEX IS A RANKING OF CARBOHYDRATE FOODS BASED ON THEIR IMMEDIATE EFFECT ON BLOOD SUGAR LEVELS.

■

Chapter 5

SOURCES OF CARBOHYDRATE

*A*t the beginning of this book we explained that carbohydrate is the fuel our bodies like best. Carbohydrate is important for children because it gives them the energy they need every day to play, study and take part in sports.

Breads and cereals, vegetables and fruits are all sources of carbohydrate. Milk products also contain carbohydrate in the form of milk sugar, or lactose, which is the first carbohydrate we consume as babies.

Some foods contain a large amount of carbohydrate (cereals, potatoes and legumes are good examples), while other foods, such as carrots and broccoli and salad vegetables, are very dilute sources and don't provide nearly enough carbohydrate for our high carbohydrate diet. So, as nutritious as salads can be, they aren't meals on their own and need to be complemented with a carbohydrate food such as whole grain bread or pasta.

Chapter 6

WHY WE NEED MORE CARBOHYDRATE

Most experts agree that breakfast, lunch, dinner and in-between snack foods should be low in fat and high in carbohydrate. And when it comes to choosing the best fuel for vigorous and extended physical activity—whether it's sports or play—again, carbohydrate is the best choice. Studies show that a balanced carbohydrate meal enhances memory and learning; in fact, children's scores on classroom tests are higher if they consume healthy carbohydrates for breakfast.

In addition, carbohydrate and fat have a reciprocal relationship in our diets: if we eat more high carbohydrate foods they tend to displace the high fat foods from our diet. And when carbohydrates (such as a breakfast of Special K, skim milk and fruit, instead of a chocolate doughnut) displace saturated and trans fats, they improve the diet's overall nutritional quality. In fact, carbohydrate should be the main source of calories in our food—not fat.

■

A HEALTHY, BALANCED DIET FOR CHILDREN CONTAINS A WIDE VARIETY OF FOODS.

■

CARBOHYDRATES AND INSULIN

The pancreas is a vital organ near the stomach, and its main job is to produce the hormone insulin. Carbohydrate stimulates the secretion of insulin more than any other component of food. The slow absorption of the carbohydrate in our food means that the pancreas doesn't have to work so hard and needs to produce less insulin. If the pancreas is overstimulated over a long period of time, it may become "exhausted" and type 2 diabetes can develop in genetically susceptible people. Even without diabetes, high insulin levels are undesirable because they increase the risk of heart disease.

Unfortunately, over time, we have begun to eat more "refined" foods and fewer "whole" foods. This new way of eating has brought with it higher blood sugar levels after a meal and higher insulin responses, as well. Though our bodies do need insulin for carbohydrate metabolism, high levels of the hormone have a profound effect on the development of many diseases. In fact, medical experts now believe that high insulin levels are one of the key factors responsible for heart disease and hypertension. Insulin influences the way we metabolize foods, determining whether we burn fat or carbohydrate to meet our energy needs and ultimately determining whether we store fat in our bodies.

Chapter 7

THE GLYCEMIC INDEX: SOME BACKGROUND

The glycemic index of foods is simply a ranking of foods based on their immediate effect on blood sugar levels. To make a fair comparison, all foods are compared with a reference food such as pure glucose and are tested in equivalent carbohydrate amounts.

Today we know the glycemic index of hundreds of different food items—both generic and name-brand—that have been tested following a standardized testing method. The tables on pages 128-142 give the glycemic index of a range of common foods, including many tested at the University of Toronto and the University of Sydney.

HOW THE GLYCEMIC INDEX CAME TO BE

The glycemic index concept was first developed in 1981 by a team of scientists led by Dr. David Jenkins, a professor of nutrition at the University of Toronto, Canada, to help determine which foods were best for people with diabetes. At that time, the diet for people with diabetes was based on a system of carbohydrate exchanges or portions, which was complicated and not very logical. The carbohydrate exchange system assumed that all starchy foods produce the same effect on blood sugar levels even though some earlier studies had already proven this was not correct. Jenkins was one of the first researchers to question this assumption and to investigate how real foods behave in the bodies of real people.

Jenkins's approach attracted a great deal of attention because it was so logical and systematic. He and his colleagues had tested a large number of common foods, and some of their results were surprising. Ice cream for example, despite its sugar content, had much less effect on blood sugar than some ordinary breads. Over the next fifteen years medical researchers and scientists around the world, including the authors of this book, tested the effect of many foods on blood sugar levels and developed a new concept of classifying carbohydrates based on their glycemic index.

When we looked at the actual blood sugar responses to different foods in people we found that:

- Many complex carbohydrates, such as bread and potatoes, were actually digested and absorbed very quickly (contrary to popular opinion).
- Many sugar-containing foods were not the villains responsible for high blood sugars.

Carbohydrate foods that break down quickly during digestion have the highest G.I. values. The blood glucose, or sugar, response is fast and high. In other words the glucose in the bloodstream increases rapidly. Conversely, carbohydrates that break down slowly, releasing glucose gradually into the bloodstream, have low G.I. values. An analogy might be the popular fable of the tortoise and the hare. The hare, just like high G.I. foods, speeds away full steam ahead but loses the race to the tortoise with his slow and steady pace. Similarly, slow and steady low G.I. foods produce a smooth blood sugar curve without wild fluctuations.

For most people most of the time, the foods with low G.I. values have advantages over those with high G.I. values. To see the effect of slow and fast carbohydrate on blood sugar levels, see Figure 1.

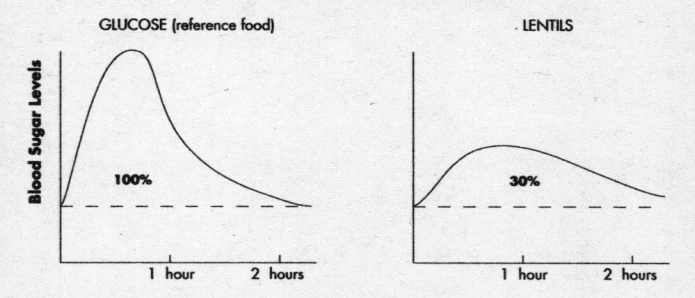

Figure 1. The effect of pure glucose (50 grams) and lentils (50 grams carbohydrate portion) on blood sugar levels.

THE GLYCEMIC INDEX IS:

- a scientifically proven guide to the actual effects of carbohydrate foods on blood sugar levels, and
- an easy and effective way to eat a healthy diet and control fluctuations in blood sugar.

THE GLYCEMIC INDEX IS A CLINICALLY PROVEN TOOL IN ITS APPLICATIONS TO DIABETES, APPETITE CONTROL AND REDUCING THE RISK OF HEART DISEASE.

Chapter 8

HOW WE MEASURE THE GLYCEMIC INDEX

The substance that produces the greatest rise in blood sugar levels is pure glucose itself. All other foods have less effect when fed in equal amounts of carbohydrate. The glycemic index of pure glucose is set at 100, and every other food is ranked on a scale from 0 to 100 according to its actual effect on blood sugar levels.

We can't predict the glycemic index of a food from its composition or the glycemic index of related foods. To test the glycemic index, we need real people and real foods. There is no easy, inexpensive substitute test. Scientists always follow standardized methods so that results from one group of people can be directly compared with those of another group.

The most important point to note is that all foods are tested in equivalent carbohydrate amounts. For example, we test 100 grams of bread (about 3½ slices of sandwich bread) because that amount contains 50 grams of carbohydrate. Likewise, 60 grams of jelly beans (containing 50 grams of carbohydrate) is compared with the reference food. We know how much carbohydrate is in a food by consulting food composition tables, the manufacturer's data or measuring it ourselves in the laboratory.

Scientists use just six steps to determine the glycemic index of a food. Simple as this may sound, it's actually quite a time consuming process. Here's how it works.

1. An amount of food containing 50 grams of carbohydrate is given to a volunteer to eat. For example, to test boiled spaghetti, the volunteer would be given 200 grams of spaghetti, which supplies 50 grams of carbohydrate (we work this out from food composition tables or by measuring the available carbohydrate)—50 grams of carbohydrate is equivalent to 3 tablespoons of pure glucose powder.
2. Over the next two hours (or three hours if the volunteer has diabetes), we take a sample of their blood every 15 minutes during the first hour and thereafter every 30 minutes. The blood sugar level of these blood samples is measured in the laboratory and recorded.
3. The blood sugar level is plotted on a graph and the area under the curve is calculated using a computer program (Figure 2).
4. The volunteer's response to spaghetti (or whatever food is being tested) is compared with his or her blood sugar response to 50 grams of

pure glucose (the reference food).

5. The reference food is tested on two or three separate occasions and an average value is calculated. This is done to reduce the effect of day-to-day variation in blood sugar responses.
6. The average glycemic index found in 8 to 10 people is the glycemic index of that food.

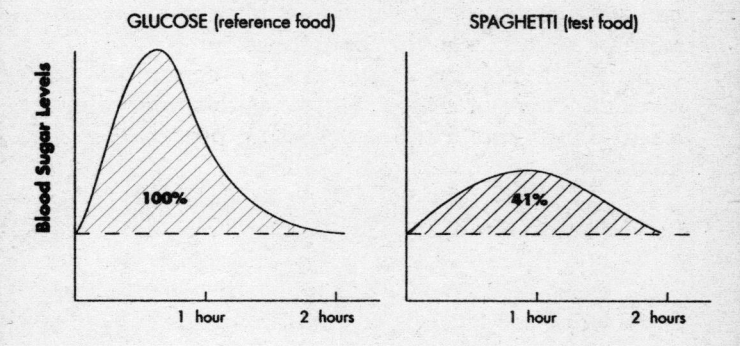

Figure 2.

Part 2

THE GLYCEMIC INDEX AND YOUR CHILD

LOW G.I. DIETS FOR CHILDREN

WHO BENEFITS FROM LOW G.I. FOODS?

THE FOOD PYRAMID FOR CHILDREN

BLOOD SUGAR AND EXERCISE

BLOOD SUGAR GUIDELINES

HANDLING LOW BLOOD SUGAR

SICK DAY HYPOGLYCEMIA

Chapter 9

LOW G.I. DIETS FOR CHILDREN

*I*t's easy to incorporate low G.I. foods into a child's diet and rewarding to watch them reap the benefits. It usually just means making a few substitutions, such as those shown on page 29. Ideally, you should aim to swap at least half of the high G.I. foods that you give children for low G.I. choices. For example, you could change the type of bread or breakfast cereal your child eats and serve pasta or legumes more often. And don't forget milk and dairy foods.

Remember that it isn't necessary to serve children only low G.I. foods. On the contrary, meals usually consist of a variety of foods, and eating a low G.I. food with a high G.I. food produces an intermediate G.I. meal. Here are three ways to make serving low G.I. foods easier:

- Become familiar with the different types of low G.I. choices available.
- Have low G.I. foods available in the pantry and refrigerator.
- Experiment with new foods and recipes.

■

TRY TO INCLUDE AT LEAST ONE LOW G.I. FOOD PER MEAL PER DAY.

■

SUBSTITUTING LOW G.I. FOR HIGH G.I. FOODS

High G.I. Food	Low G.I. Alternative
Bread; whole wheat or white	Bread containing lots of "grainy bits" that is dense, heavy and usually dark, such as 100% stoneground whole wheat, wholegrain pumpernickel and sourdough rye
Most processed breakfast cereals, such as Corn Flakes, Rice/Corn Chex, Rice Krispies, Crispix and Shredded Wheat	Unrefined cereals such as rolled oats or muesli or a low G.I. processed cereal such as All Bran and Special K
Crackers, such as saltines, Ritz, Wheatables and rice cakes; cookies such as sugar wafers, Snackwells and Oreos	Crackers such as WASA, Ry Krisp, Kavli and Ryvita; cookies such as graham crackers, oatmeal, Social Tea and Lorna Doone
Most cakes and	Muffins made with fruit, oats and 100% whole wheat flour
Tropical fruits such as bananas, pineapple, watermelon and raisins	Temperate climate fruits such as apples, pears, peaches, nectarines, all berries and grapes
White potatoes, baked or mashed	Baby new potatoes, sweet potatoes, corn, pasta and legumes
Short grain or "sticky" rice	Uncle Ben's converted rice or any other long grain, Basmati or brown rice

Chapter 10

WHO BENEFITS FROM LOW G.I. FOODS?

We all do! The slow digestion and gradual rise and fall in blood sugar levels after eating a low G.I. food reduces the secretion of the hormone insulin into the blood. High insulin levels are undesirable because they increase our risk of heart disease, diabetes and obesity. Reducing this risk is why low G.I. foods benefit everyone—people with and without diabetes. These facts are no exaggeration: They're confirmed by many studies published in prestigious journals around the world.

G.I. VALUE RANGES

Low G.I. foods = below 55
Intermediate G.I. foods = between 55 and 70
High G.I. foods = greater than 70

LOW G.I./HIGH G.I. CHOICES

A food is neither good nor bad based on its glycemic index. For example, if a food is high in fat, it's not a good idea to eat it regularly just because it has a low G.I. value. By the same token, we shouldn't demonize low fat, high G.I. foods like some types of potatoes. The truth is, eating a potato is far better than eating a food loaded with saturated fat, even if its glycemic index is low.

■

CONSIDER THE G.I. VALUE OF A FOOD IN CONJUNCTION WITH ITS FAT, FIBER AND SALT CONTENT — NOT BY ITSELF.

■

FOOD FOR THOUGHT

Children have different nutritional requirements at different ages. That's why, if you have a child with diabetes, you'll need to review and adjust her diet with the help of a dietitian.

Chapter 11

THE FOOD PYRAMID FOR CHILDREN

*S*chool-age children have changing energy needs due to their growth rate, body size and physical activity level. All children need at least the minimum number of servings from each of the five food groups every day. Older, larger and more active children will require the maximum number of servings, which will give their bodies the 1,800 to 2,200 calories they require for proper growth and good health.

CHILDREN WITH TYPE 1 DIABETES

THE FOOD PYRAMID FOR CHILDREN

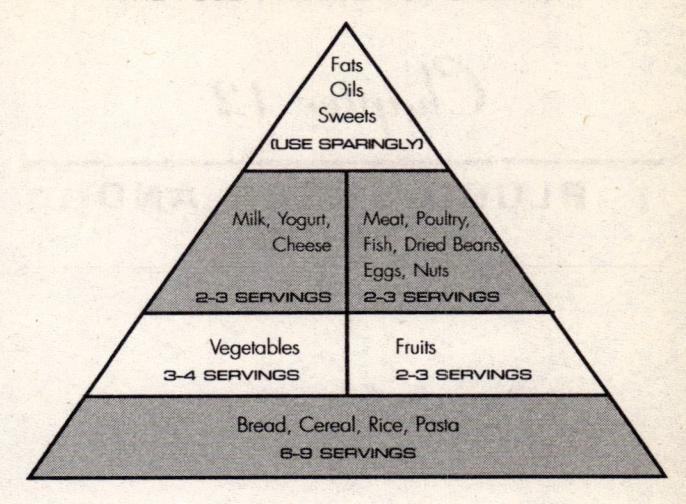

- Fats, Oils, Sweets (USE SPARINGLY)
- Milk, Yogurt, Cheese — 2-3 SERVINGS
- Meat, Poultry, Fish, Dried Beans, Eggs, Nuts — 2-3 SERVINGS
- Vegetables — 3-4 SERVINGS
- Fruits — 2-3 SERVINGS
- Bread, Cereal, Rice, Pasta — 6-9 SERVINGS

IS YOUR CHILD GETTING ENOUGH WATER?

Water Requirements	Ounces/Lb./Day
0– 3 mos.	1.2 – 2.5
4 – 6 mos.	2.0 – 2.3
7 –12 mos.	1.8 – 2.0
1 year	1.8 – 2.0
2 years	1.7 – 1.9
6 years	1.4 – 1.3

■

IF CHILDREN LEARN TO COMBINE REGULAR PHYSICAL ACTIVITY WITH HEALTHY LOW G.I. EATING EARLY IN THEIR LIVES, THEY WILL BE DEVELOPING HEALTHY LIFESTYLE HABITS THAT MAY CONTINUE INTO ADULTHOOD.

■

Chapter 12

BLOOD SUGAR AND EXERCISE

Good health, a reasonable body weight and good blood sugar levels are all easier to achieve if children exercise, because their insulin will work better.

If they get additional exercise or take part in activities outside their normal routine, children may need to eat extra carbohydrates as a precaution to prevent their blood sugar levels from dropping too low. Just how much extra carbohydrate they'll need will depend on their fitness level, the type and length of activity and the amount of effort they're expending. As a rough guide, one extra serving of carbohydrate is suggested for every hour of strenuous activity. Generally, the more strenuous and the longer the duration of the exercise, the more additional carbohydrate they will require.

Your child's usual insulin dose and food intake covers normal play activities—even quite strenuous ones.

APPROPRIATE BLOOD SUGAR LEVELS

If your child's blood sugar is less than 180 mg/dl before exercise, she may need to eat extra carbohydrates before, during and after exercise to prevent hypoglycemia. (Mg/dl is a unit of measurement for the concentration of sugar in a given quantity of blood.)

If your child's blood sugar is more than 270 mg/dl and ketones are present in her urine before exercise, ask her to postpone exercise until her overall control has improved. Otherwise, exercise may actually increase her blood sugar level further. (Ketones are a product of fat breakdown that occurs when there isn't enough insulin available. Without adequate insulin, the body isn't able to use its preferred fuel—glucose—so it uses fat instead.)

Since everyone responds to exercise differently, your child may need to eat extra carbohydrates before and/or during and/or after exercise, and the quantity she needs may also vary.

You and your child will learn from experience what works best for her; at first, monitoring her blood sugar before, during and after exercise will give both of you the best indication of how her body responds.

SUSTAINING BLOOD SUGAR LEVELS DURING EXERCISE

- If children eat immediately before exercising, they should select foods with a high glycemic index, such as sugar wafers, candy, granola bars or a white bread sandwich.

- When kids eat 1 or 2 hours before exercising, they should choose low G.I. foods such as yogurt, a sandwich made from low G.I. bread, low G.I. cereals, low G.I. fruits or milkshakes.
- If children need to eat during prolonged exercise (over an hour), they need to choose foods with a high glycemic index that they can eat on the run. Liquids—sports drinks—may be best because they meet fuel and fluid requirements at the same time.
- If kids eat between events throughout the day (such as at bike races or a day at the beach) they should eat a combination of low and high G.I. foods. It is generally appropriate to decrease the usual insulin dose by 10 percent as well, so that they don't need to eat too much food.
- If children require additional foods to restore blood sugar levels after exercise, they should choose high G.I. foods such as rice cakes, white bread, watermelon or a high G.I. cereal such as Rice Krispies or corn flakes. They need to drink plenty of water, too, or select high G.I. fluids to meet both carbohydrate and fluid needs at the same time.

■

EXERCISE MEANS BEING ACTIVE EVERY DAY — WHETHER IT'S PLAYING A SPORT, TAKING PART IN AN ACTIVE HOBBY OR WALKING THE DOG AFTER SCHOOL.

■

Chapter 13

BLOOD SUGAR GUIDELINES

In order to maintain a healthy weight, children of all ages need to strike a balance between eating a well-balanced diet based on low G.I. foods and getting enough exercise. Low G.I. foods not only help your child maintain blood sugar control, but they're also more sustaining and can make her feel fuller longer, compared with foods with a high G.I. value.

To make sure that they eat well and exercise regularly, all kids should:

- limit high fat foods such as chocolate, chips, cookies, fried foods, burgers, potato chips, and cake.

- keep in contact with their health professional. As they lose weight, their diabetes team should review their insulin doses.
- do something active everyday. Increasing physical activity doesn't have to mean vigorous exercise: It simply means spending less time lying around.
- incorporate exercise into their daily routine. There are lots of options, from team sports to aerobics classes, swimming or gym workouts. If youngsters want to do something less structured, they can walk, jog, cycle, or go inline skating.

■

BEING MORE ACTIVE MAKES KIDS LOOK BETTER AND FEEL BETTER. HONEST!

■

FOOD FOR THOUGHT

Studies show that people who take more than 12,500 steps a day don't gain weight over the long term, no matter what they eat. Children can measure how many steps they take in a single day by using a pedometer.

Chapter 14

HANDLING LOW BLOOD SUGAR

*H*ypoglycemia occurs when there are low levels of sugar in the blood, usually below 55 to 70 mg/dl.

Low blood sugar may be caused by:

- taking too much insulin;
- exercising vigorously without eating extra carbohydrate;
- missing or delaying meals; or
- not eating an adequate amount of carbohydrate food.

How children feel when their blood sugar is low varies from child to child. Common symptoms are excessive sweating, tiredness, drowsiness, irritability, dizziness, shaking, headache, and blurred vision.

■

LEARN THE SIGNS OF LOW BLOOD SUGAR AND ACT QUICKLY. IF THESE DIPS HAPPEN OFTEN, CONTACT YOUR DOCTOR OR DIABETES EDUCATOR SO THEY CAN REVIEW YOUR CHILD'S INSULIN DOSE AND DIET.

■

WHAT TO DO ABOUT LOW BLOOD SUGAR

To combat hypoglycemia, your child should:

- eat a quickly absorbed (high G.I.) carbohydrate food that's easy to eat or drink (jellybeans, regular soda, Gatorade, orange juice). The food will immediately increase blood sugar levels. If she sees no improvement, your child should eat more high G.I. food after five minutes have passed.
- follow the above guideline by eating an intermediate or low G.I. carbohydrate food (bread, cookies, fruit, milk) ten to fifteen minutes after to a) ensure that her blood sugar level remains within the normal range longer and b) prevent the hypo from recurring.
- always carry high G.I. foods or glucose tablets to treat hypoglycemia.
- remember that the extra foods she eats for low blood sugar are *extra* and should not be subtracted from her next meal or snack.
- try to determine why the hypoglycemia occurred, in order to help prevent it from happening again. Most hypoglycemic episodes are preventable but some occur for no apparent reason.

> **DON'T LEAVE SOMEONE WITH HYPOGLYCEMIA UNATTENDED UNTIL THEY ARE FEELING BETTER.**

COPING WITH LOW BLOOD SUGAR AT NIGHT

Hypoglycemia can occur at night. Most of the time, though, children wake when they're experiencing low blood sugar, or at least they become restless enough that their parents wake up. Sometimes, however, children sleep soundly through a blood sugar drop and the body self-corrects and over-compensates, which shows up as a high blood sugar reading the next morning.

MINIMIZING THE RISK OF NIGHT-TIME HYPOGLYCEMIA

You can help to reduce the risk of low blood sugar at night by asking your child to:

- eat a low G.I. bedtime snack (such as a glass of milk or no-sugar-added hot chocolate and three Social Tea biscuits or one slice of toast), even if the evening blood sugar test is high.
- never skip the bedtime snack, even if the evening blood sugar test is high.
- test blood sugar levels before bed, once your doctor has helped you determine her appropriate pre-bed level. Your child may need some extra carbohydrate.

FOOD FOR THOUGHT

Have a Registered Dietitian evaluate your child's normal calorie intake to make sure that it's adequate. Because children's energy needs vary with age and physical activity levels, an ongoing nutritional assessment can help with blood sugar control.

Chapter 15

SICK DAY HYPOGLYCEMIA

*H*aving a sick child can be hard enough, but a sick child with diabetes means that you need to be extra vigilant about blood sugar levels and appetite. Here are some guidelines.

IF BLOOD SUGAR READINGS ARE GREATER THAN 270 MG/DL:

Serve your child low calorie fluids such as water or decaffeinated diet drinks. You may also offer slightly smaller portions of carbohydrate foods while the sugar remains high since you're monitoring the readings more frequently. Don't omit carbohydrate foods altogether.

IF BLOOD SUGAR READINGS ARE LESS THAN 270 MG/DL:

Serve your child some form of carbohydrate. Choosing foods from the intermediate G.I. range (or combining low G.I. foods with high G.I. foods) will help sustain blood sugar levels while your child has a reduced appetite. Try serving:

plain toast	ice cream	stewed fruit
dry crackers	milkshakes	fruit juices
cookies	soup	potato chips

If your child's appetite is poor, he should frequently eat or sip intermediate to high G.I. foods. (It may be easier for your child to eat smaller amounts more often.) Try offering these foods:

a sweetened soft drink	sweetened jelly	jellybeans	Jello
Gatorade	ices or ice pops	lollipops	pudding

If your child has diarrhea associated with gastroenteritis, you *must* dilute sweet fluids with water (one part water to one part soft drink). Avoid serving your child full-strength sweet fluid, since that may actually worsen the diarrhea. Some salty fluids such as soup broths or tomato juice may also help your child rehydrate.

FOOD FOR THOUGHT

Occasionally check your child's blood sugar readings at 2:00 or 3:00 A.M. This early-morning check is especially important if your child is sick, has eaten poorly over the course of the day, has been unusually active or if you suspect nighttime hypoglycemia.

GENERAL SICK-DAY GUIDELINES

Your child is likely to get coughs and colds and all the normal childhood illnesses. Unfortunately, sickness can make diabetes hard to manage, and lack of appetite is partly to blame. It's essential to monitor blood sugars closely during an illness.

ALWAYS GIVE INSULIN

When children are sick, their liver is still producing (perhaps over-producing) glucose to maintain blood sugar levels. Insulin is essential in order to manage this output. To maintain blood glucose control:

- Monitor blood sugar levels every 2 hours.
- Test for ketones in the urine throughout the day. Your child may need extra insulin if ketones are present.
- Continue to serve some form of carbohydrates and make sure your child drinks plenty of fluids.

■

IF YOU'RE EVER IN DOUBT WHEN CARING FOR A SICK CHILD WITH DIABETES, CALL YOUR DIABETES DOCTOR OR EDUCATOR FOR ADDITIONAL ADVICE.

■

Part 3

FOOD BASICS

CEREALS AND GRAIN FOODS

VEGETABLES

FRUIT

DAIRY FOODS

MEAT AND MEAT ALTERNATIVES

FATS AND OILS

SUGAR

Chapter 16

CEREALS AND GRAIN FOODS

Today, cereal and grains are major sources of energy and protein for people all over the world, but they weren't part of the diet that humankind evolved on millions of years ago. As human populations grew, resources of mammals, fish and birds became depleted. It's only been over the last 10,000 years that we've begun to rely more on cereals for food—with consequent developments in processing.

Unprocessed cereals and grains are naturally slowly digested foods. In early times, they were roughly ground between stones, which broke the outer seed husk but left much of the grain intact and produced a coarse meal. Today, cereal processing includes milling the grain into a fine flour, then popping, toasting, flaking and extrusion cooking to make cakes, breads, cookies, snack products and breakfast cereals.

One of the nutritional implications of this dietary change has been an increase in the G.I. value, because modern processing methods transform the low G.I. carbohydrate of cereal grains to high G.I. foods. In other words, because of the processing (or refinement) of whole grains, our bodies have much less work to do to digest them into blood sugar (glucose) and dump them into the bloodstream.

To help your child eat a low G.I. diet, serve less-processed cereal products and whole grain cereals. Hint: The higher the fiber content, the more intact the grains are. Aim for 5 grams of fiber or more per serving.

PASTA

Most children love pasta. And not only is it good to eat, it's good to eat it often because whether you choose penne or spaghetti or fettuccine, you are choosing one of nature's naturally low G.I. foods.

Most pasta is made from semolina (finely cracked wheat), which is milled from very hard wheat with a high protein content. A stiff dough, made by mixing the semolina with water, is forced through a die and dried. There is very little disruption of the starch granule during this process and the strong protein-starch interactions inhibit starch gelatinization. The dense consistency also makes the pasta resistant to disruption in the small intestine and contributes to the final low glycemic index—even pasta made from fine flour (instead of semolina) has a relatively low glycemic index. There's some evidence that thicker pasta has a lower glycemic index than thin types because of its dense consistency and perhaps because it cooks more slowly. (It's also less likely to be overcooked.) The addition of egg to fresh pasta lowers the G.I. value by increasing the protein content: Higher protein levels slow stomach emptying, because only about 60 percent of the protein gets broken down; the rest goes into storage as fat.

Italians eat their pasta "al dente" which literally means "to the tooth." It must be slightly firm and offer some resistance when you're chewing it. Not only does al dente pasta taste better than soft, soggy pasta, but it also has a lower G.I. value, because overcooking pasta increases starch gelatinization (or swelling) and boosts its glycemic index.

> *OUR BOOKS THE GLUCOSE REVOLUTION AND THE GLUCOSE REVOLUTION LIFE PLAN HAVE MANY RECIPES THAT YOUR WHOLE FAMILY WILL ENJOY.*

RICE

Rice is an ideal accompaniment to spicy foods. Milling rice removes the bran and germ, which results in a considerable nutrient loss. Brown rice is a better source of B vitamins, minerals and fiber; be sure to vary your family's diet to include both brown and white rice. And look for other lower G.I. rices, including Uncle Ben's converted or Basmati rice, in your supermarket.

BREAD

One of the most important changes you can make to lower the G.I. value of your children's diet is to choose a low G.I. bread when making toast, sandwiches or snacks.

Choose dense breads that contain a lot of whole grains: If the fibrous seed coat of cereal grains is intact it acts as a physical barrier to slow down starch digestion. Pumpernickel is a true whole grain bread—it's made from whole rye grains.

Other low G.I. breads include sourdough and stone ground flour breads (types that don't contain any enriched wheat flour). The acids in sourdough breads may reduce the glycemic index—the acids that result from fermentation of the starch and sugars are believed to lower G.I. values by slowing down stomach emptying. To add more bread to your child's meals, read our sandwich suggestions for snacks and school lunches on pages 99 and 108.

If you're making your own bread, you can add your own G.I. lowering ingredients, such as linseed, flaxseed, rolled oats, cornmeal, oat bran, barley meal, cracked wheat and wheat berries.

Chapter 17

VEGETABLES

Your children can eat most vegetables without thinking about their glycemic index. Most are so low in carbohydrate that they have no measurable effect on blood sugar levels, but they still provide valuable amounts of fiber, vitamins and minerals. Higher carbohydrate vegetables include potato, sweet potato, corn and peas. Among these, corn and sweet potato are the lower G.I. choices. Pumpkin, carrots, peas, and beets contain some carbohydrate but a half-cup serving contains so little that these foods don't raise blood sugar levels significantly.

Salad vegetables such as tomatoes, lettuce, cucumber, peppers, and onions also have so little carbohydrate that it's impossible to test their glycemic index values. In generous serving sizes, they won't have any effect on blood sugars. Think of them as "free" foods that are full of healthful micronutrients.

Chapter 18

FRUIT

Not only does fruit make an ideal snack, you can transform it into a tasty-sweet dessert quickly and easily. Fruit contains carbohydrate, fiber, vitamins (such as vitamin C and beta-carotene) and minerals. Most fresh fruit contains vitamin C, so all of us—not just our children—should eat it every day, preferably whole, rather than as juice.

Most fruits have low G.I. values thanks to the low glycemic index of fructose (a major sugar in fruit). The presence of viscous fiber, such as pectin and acids (which may slow down stomach emptying), also help keep the glycemic index low.

- Fruits with the lowest G.I. values tend to be those grown in temperate climates, such as apples, pears, citrus, peaches, plums, cherries, and all berries.
- The more acidic the fruit, the lower its glycemic index; for example, grapefruit's glycemic index is 25.
- Tropical fruits, such as melons, pineapples and bananas, have intermediate G.I. values.

Chapter 19

DAIRY FOODS

You should encourage your children to eat dairy foods throughout their childhood and beyond. Not only are dairy foods an important source of calcium but they also have low G.I. values. Dairy foods also provide energy, protein, carbohydrate, vitamin B_2 and important fat-soluble vitamins such as vitamins A and D.

If for some reason your child is allergic to cow's milk, try a lactose-free milk or suitable calcium-fortified soy substitute (approximately 180 mg of calcium per 4 ounces). The soy drinks that we have tested have low G.I. values—similar to cow's milk. The good news is that most children will outgrow a cow's milk allergy by five years of age.

Calcium helps build and maintain strong bones and teeth and has other important nerve and muscle functions. Milk, yogurt, ice cream, pudding, and custard are all excellent low G.I. sources of calcium. Cheese, although a good source of calcium, is considered a source of protein rather than carbohydrate, and contains no lactose.

Chapter 20

MEAT AND MEAT ALTERNATIVES

*P*roteins are the body's building blocks, so we need to eat a variety of protein foods from animal or plant sources to create, maintain and renew our body cells. Children and teenagers, because they are growing, need more protein in relation to their body weight than adults do because they are building new body cells.

- Red meat, chicken, pork and fish are important sources of protein and micronutrients such as iron. They don't contain carbohydrate so they don't have a G.I. value. Choose lean meats where possible; there are now many trim cuts available. Serve *infrequently* such fatty processed meats as sausage, frankfurters, chicken nuggets, and salami.

- Include fish in the family meals at least once a week, especially tuna or salmon, which are high in heart-healthy omega-3 essential fatty acids.
- Legumes such as split peas, baked beans, and lentils, provide protein, vitamin B and iron, as does meat, but legumes are also excellent low G.I. sources of carbohydrate. Try to incorporate them in family meals at least once a week.

NATURAL PEANUT BUTTER

Natural peanut butter is a high protein, nutrient-dense food. It contains fiber, iron and heart-healthy monounsaturated fat. Peanut butter and all-fruit jelly on whole grain bread is a great breakfast, lunch or snack that requires little time or skill to prepare! And just for variety, you can try other nut butters, such as cashew, almond and soy.

Chapter 21

FATS AND OILS

Although fat doesn't directly affect blood sugar levels, it isn't something that you can ignore. The fat that children (and all of us) eat affects their body weight, cholesterol levels, risk of diabetic complications and odds of developing poor health from everyday diseases such as obesity, heart disease and even cancer.

Although a low fat diet is *not recommended* for very young children, once a child is older than five, it's fine for them to eat low fat products. If your child is overweight, limiting fat intake will likely help, but you should only do this under the guidance of a registered dietitian.

It's important to consider what type of fat your child eats. For example, polyunsaturated fats such as margarine and vegetable oils, and monounsaturated fats such as olive and canola oils are preferable to saturated fats such as butter and fatty meats. In fact, we all should limit our saturated fat intake. It's particularly important for children to avoid saturated fat because the changes in blood vessels that lead to heart disease begin in childhood. You'll find a list of high fat foods on this page.

FOOD FOR THOUGHT

The omega-3 fats found in fish are important sources of healthy fat for adults as well as children, so try to serve fish, such as salmon and white albacore tuna, regularly.

HIGH FAT FOODS TO WATCH OUT FOR:

Butter
Cakes, cookies
Cheese
Chicken nuggets
Whole milk (Children under age two should be given whole milk.)
Corn chips
Creamy soups, sauces and desserts
Doughnuts
French fries
Ice-creams
Most milkshakes
Pastries
Pies
Pizza with meat and cheese toppings
Potato chips
Sausages
Solid cooking fats and cooking margarines; white fat on beef, lamb, pork, vegetable shortening

Chapter 22

SUGAR

Children naturally enjoy sweet foods. Sweetness is not a learned taste; in fact it could be said that we're all born with "a sweet tooth." Not only is our first food—breast milk—sweet, but also infants smile when offered a sweet solution, as they reject sour and bitter tastes.

Did you know that a balanced diet should include some fat and sugar? Studies over the past decade have found that high sugar diets are no less nutritious than diets containing lower amounts of sugar: When we restrict sugar, we frequently eat more fat, and the most popular fatty foods are poor sources of nutrients. In some cases, high sugar diets may have higher micronutrient contents, because sugar is often used to sweeten some very nutritious foods, such as yogurt, breakfast cereals and milk.

Today, glycemic index researchers have tested hundreds of real foods on real people, and the results are surprising: Sugar is not the dietary demon that it was once made out to be. Many Americans, though, eat far too much of it. Sixteen percent of our average daily caloric intake comes from sweeteners (health experts recommend six to ten percent). That's why you need to look at your child's diet and adjust her sugar intake accordingly. Your child can enjoy sugar and foods containing sugar *in moderation* as part of a balanced low G.I. diet.

FOOD FOR THOUGHT

It's not a good idea for children—or any of us—to eat an excess of artificially sweetened products. Many of these products, such as diet sodas and sugar-free candies and sweets, are simply flavored fillers and provide few, if any, nutrients. It is nutritionally unwise to allow children to fill up on calorie-free, nutrient-*free* foods—serve them nutrient-*packed* foods instead.

WHAT EXACTLY IS "MODERATE INTAKE"?

A moderate intake of refined sugar for a child is between 7 to 12 teaspoons a day. Keep in mind that we're talking about the sugar found in foods, such as all non-diet soft drinks, breakfast cereals, candy, ice cream, cookies, jelly and syrups. Staying within this amount of sugar can make your child's diet more enjoyable without compromising her blood sugar control.

CHILDREN WITH TYPE 1 DIABETES

A MODERATE-SUGAR MENU

This child's menu provides 45 grams of refined sugar (about 3 ½ tablespoons) and 1,700 calories (29 percent of energy from fat, 54 percent from carbohydrate and 17 percent from protein).

Breakfast
- ½ cup Special K with 6 ozs. 1% milk
- ½ cup strawberries
- 1 teaspoon sugar

Mid-morning snack
- 4 ozs. unsweetened applesauce
- 15 Teddy Grahams

Lunch
- Ham and cheese sandwich on multigrain bread with lettuce and tomato
- 1 cup grapes
- 2 Chips Ahoy chocolate chip cookies

After-school snack
- 6 ozs. 1% milk
- 6 Social Tea biscuits

Dinner
- 1 cup spaghetti with ½ cup meat sauce
- ½ cup steamed French cut green beans
- ½ cup Snack Pack tapioca pudding

Bedtime snack
- 1 slice cinnamon raisin toast with butter or margarine
- 4 ozs. 1% milk

FAST-ACTING CARBOHYDRATES

It is absolutely essential to serve refined sugars or "fast-acting" carbohydrates in these situations:

- During periods of hypoglycemia (low blood sugar levels);
- When your child is ill and has little or no appetite;
- Immediately before exercise or strenuous activity; and
- As a treat or on a special occasion.

FOOD FOR THOUGHT

"Carbohydrate modified" sugar alcohols, such as sorbitol, mannitol and xylitol, often produce a laxative effect if you eat too much of them.

Part 4

AGE-SPECIFIC INFORMATION FOR DIABETIC CHILDREN

BABIES

TODDLERS AND PRE-SCHOOLERS

SCHOOL-AGE CHILDREN

TEENAGERS

THE FOOD PYRAMID FOR ADOLESCENTS AND TEENAGERS

Chapter 23

BABIES

Babies with diabetes should be breastfed if possible. Although infants should dictate how much they eat, you should monitor their blood sugars routinely. If it's not possible to breastfeed, offer your baby an infant formula at least every three to four hours.

Until your baby is twelve months old, milk should be her main drink. When your baby is about seven months old, you can introduce whole cows' milk in small quantities as custard, pudding, yogurt or on cereal. From twelve months, when your baby is eating a varied diet, you can give her whole cows' milk as her main drink. Encourage your baby to eat dairy foods because they're an important source of calcium and have low G.I. values—a big advantage when you're trying to optimize your baby's blood sugar control.

You can begin introducing your child to solids (including low G.I. foods) anytime from five to six months—when your baby is ready. By twelve months she should be enjoying the family meal with you and drinking whole cows' milk from a cup. (Your whole family can enjoy delicious low G.I. meals: Our books *The Glucose Revolution* and *The Glucose Revolution Life Plan* contain hundreds of recipes, and meal and snack ideas that your whole family will enjoy.)

FOOD FOR THOUGHT

A word about toddler tantrums

Tantrums are common among independent toddlers. But sometimes it's difficult to determine whether a toddler is irritable because of hypoglycemia or the "terrible twos." When in doubt, remember that it's potentially more dangerous *not* to treat hypoglycemia in a young child.

CHILDREN WITH TYPE 1 DIABETES

RECOMMENDED DAILY QUANTITIES OF FOOD IN BABY'S FIRST YEAR

Age in months	Food Group	Food	Suggested daily amount
5–6	Dairy	Breast milk or infant formula	On demand (maximum intake 36 ozs. in 24 hours)
	Grains	Pureed/strained iron-fortified cereal: Rice, barley or oatmeal	Start with 1 tablespoon per feeding and gradually increase to 3 tablespoons/ 2 servings a day
7–9	Dairy	Breat milk or infant formula	On demand (maximum intake 36 ozs. in 24 hours)
	Grains	Pureed/strained iron-fortified cereal: rice, barley or oatmeal, Cream of Wheat, farina. Add dry low G.I. toast and crackers (not cookies)	1–3 tablespoons/ 2 servings a day
	Vegetables	Strained carrots, green beans, green peas, squash, sweet potatoes	Start with 1 tablespoon per feeding, increase to 2 tablespoons per feeding twice a day. Add one new food every 5–6 days
	Fruit	Start fruits after vegetables Single strained fruit (pear, peaches) or mashed banana; Unsweetened fruit juice in a cup	2–3 tablespoons/ 2 servings a day
	Meat	Start meats after vegetables and fruits	2 tablespoons per feeding/1–2 serving a day

Age in months	Food Group	Food	Suggested daily amount
7–9	Meat	Strained beef, liver, veal, turkey, chicken, lamb, or pork	servings a day
10–12	Dairy	Breast milk or infant formula. May also add soft cheese, pudding and custard occasionally	On demand (maximum intake intake 36 ozs. in 24 hours) from a bottle or cup
	Grains	Continue with high iron cereals and low G.I. breads. Avoid cookies and cakes	½ cup/2 servings a day
	Vegetables	Begin slowly to increase variety. All vegetables should be cooked; may be mashed or left whole in small soft pieces. Vegetables may be spoon-fed or eaten as finger foods.	¼ cup/2 servings a day
	Fruit	Gradually increase variety. Avoid all fruits with seeds, pits, or thick skins	3 servings a day (limit fruit juice to 4 ozs. per day)
	High Protein Foods	In addition to previously mentioned choices—all of which should be appropriately cooked, ground, pureed, mashed, or flaked; cooked egg yolk (no whites) and fish may also be offered.	1–2 servings a day

Source: *Manual for Clinical Dietetics*, Fifth Edition, Chicago: The American Dietetic Association, 1996.

*It is recommended to prepare all the above listed foods at home and to avoid commercially prepared baby foods. Home preparation ensures greater nutritive value.

CHILDREN WITH TYPE 1 DIABETES

FOOD FOR THOUGHT

When possible, avoid feeding your children junior baby foods because of their limited nutritive value, limited variety and high price.

Here is a list of foods that you *should not* feed infants less than one year old:

- Whole, low fat, nonfat or evaporated cows' milk
- Cereal in a bottle
- Cereal-egg-meat mixtures in jars
- Cookies, cakes or sweet breads
- Vegetables seasoned with fat, salt, sugar or other seasonings
- Strong-flavored vegetables
- Whole kernel corn
- Infant or homemade desserts, pies or honey-fruit mixtures
- Fruits with seeds, pits or thick skins
- Vegetable-meat or pasta-meat combinations
- Fatback, bacon
- Pork, sausages
- Broth, gravy
- Candy, nuts or popcorn
- Fried foods
- Carbonated and sweetened beverages
- Regular tea

Chapter 24

TODDLERS AND PRE-SCHOOLERS

Although toddlers like to explore and show their independence, they are still too young to understand their dietary needs. This lack of understanding can sometimes cause difficulties when children are with their friends, at playgroup or when grown-ups "spoil" them with too many treats. Among toddlers and pre-schoolers, picky eating and food fads are also common.

Toddlers don't eat much, simply because they don't need to eat much. Refusing food is also a way for them to express their new-found independence. That's why it's important not to fuss or pay her special attention, since a hungry toddler will never starve.

The trouble is, children with diabetes need to eat carbohydrates regularly to prevent hypoglycemia, so parents naturally become anxious. But bribing, bullying and fussing usually only make matters worse. The best way to cope with food refusal is to try to avoid the whole situation in the first place. Allow your toddler to graze throughout the day according to her appetite rather than expecting her to eat meals at set times. Here are some other strategies to help defuse the situation:

Don't panic. Don't resort to circus tricks, since this may give your child the impression that if she refuses food, she'll get lots of attention.

Bargain calmly. Try to get the carbohydrate foods in first: "You can leave your egg if you eat your toast."

Try substituting. Substitute food that your toddler is refusing with another carbohydrate food that you know she likes. Offer only one alternative food each time though, or you could be starting a never-ending game of choices. Don't offer indulgent snack foods as alternatives.

Try finger foods and snacks. If your toddler still refuses to eat, leave finger foods (such as fruit pieces, crackers or finger sandwiches) nearby so she can nibble as she plays.

Try distraction. Sitting your toddler on your lap and reading her a book can be a good distraction and may encourage her to eat.

Be prepared for low blood sugar. When all else fails, be prepared for hypoglycemia. If that happens, serve Gatorade or a soft drink. Just don't treat the low blood sugar with jelly beans or candy: Your child may interpret candy as a reward for not eating her meal, which would reinforce her food refusals.

WHEN YOUR CHILD CONTINUES TO REFUSE FOOD

You may need to reduce your child's insulin dose temporarily to minimize the risk of hypoglycemia and to reduce her tension and anxiety until she begins to eat more.

Remember, there's no single food that your toddler must eat. Encourage her to enjoy exploring new tastes and sensations in unchallenged and comfortable surroundings.

Try introducing new foods together with familiar foods that your toddler likes. Try offering them at several different meals and with other children who like to eat those foods. Never force her to eat, since too much pressure may only encourage her to refuse food. Respect your toddler's wishes if she says that she's full. Encourage her during mealtime so that she feels confident about trying new tastes.

RECOMMENDED DAILY QUANTITIES OF FOOD FOR TODDLERS AND PRE-SCHOOLERS

Food Group	Recommended Daily Servings	Recommended Serving Sizes 1–3 yrs.	4–5 yrs.
Bread (low G.I.)		¼–½ slice	1 slice
Crackers (low G.I.)	≥ 6	2–3	4–6
Dry cereal (low G.I.)		¼–⅓ cup	½ cup
Cooked cereal, rice, pasta (low G.I.)		¼–⅓ cup	⅓ cup
Fruits and vegetables (low G.I.)	≥ 5	¼–⅓ cup ½ piece	¼–½ cup ½ piece
Milk, yogurt	≥ 3	½ cup (4 ozs.)	¾ cup (6 ozs.)
Lean meat, fish, poultry		1–2 ozs.	2–3 ozs.
Cheese	≥ 2	½ oz.	¾ oz.
Eggs		1	1
Dried peas, beans	1–3 Tbsp.	1–3 Tbsp.	
Margarine, butter, oil	3–4	1 tsp.	1 tsp.

Source: *Manual for Clinical Dietetics*, Fifth Edition, Chicago: The American Dietetic Association, 1996.

Chapter 25

SCHOOL-AGE CHILDREN

Once they're at school, children with diabetes usually become more independent and start taking some responsibility for their own diabetes care. You should encourage this responsibility, although you should still continue to support and supervise your child. The majority of diabetic primary school children take two injections per day, pre-breakfast and pre-dinner. Since blood testing during the school day usually isn't required, children with diabetes can attend school without having to deal with the hassles of injections and finger pricks. Teachers, the school nurse and other school staff should be fully educated and updated on your child's diabetes status.

LUNCH BOX IDEAS

At school, children compare lunch boxes and start trading and swapping what's inside. It's important that your child understand her diet and the carbohydrates she eats so that she can make appropriate lunch swaps. To make her more aware, involve her in preparing her school lunch. Pack enough foods to cover recess and lunch, and possibly extra for sports or after-school activities.

Try to include an interesting selection of low G.I. food choices each day and vary the contents regularly so she doesn't become bored. It's important to remember that most kids don't want to stand out from their peers, so the contents of your child's lunch box shouldn't look too different from her friends'. (For some nutritious, wholesome lunch ideas, see "The Low G.I. Lunch Box" on page 80 and "Lunches and Sandwich Fillers" on page 99.)

- Don't worry if your child selects the same foods for her lunch box everyday as long as her food choices are mainly healthy. She will let you know when she's bored and ready for more variety.
- Make sure that you pack enough carbohydrate foods each day to meet your child's needs for lunch, snacks, sports and unexpected extras. It's a good idea to consult with a registered dietitian periodically since your child's energy needs change over time.

THE LOW G.I. LUNCH BOX

When it comes to packing your child's lunch, let your imagination be your guide! Try these ideas for starters.

BREAD	+FRUIT	+DAIRY	+DRINK	+SNACKS
Be adventurous with bread choices. Include different bread varieties, rolls, crispbreads, crackers and muffins.	Include fresh fruit in season — whole, chopped, diced and sliced. Also serve unsweetened canned fruit packs (in natural juice) and dried fruits.	Include milk (plain or flavored), yogurt (natural, vanilla or flavored), and cheese.	You can vary drink choices daily; they can include milk, water, flavored seltzers or fruit juices on occasion. Freeze drinks in summer and store in your child's lunch box to keep the contents cool.	Check the list on page 108 for a wide variety of nourishing, healthy snacks to include in your child's lunch box.

HYPOGLYCEMIA AT SCHOOL

Hypoglycemia can occur at school, so make sure that your child is prepared: In fact, it's a good idea to put together a "low blood sugar box" for school, which should include some of her favorite high and low G.I. non-perishable finger foods, such as jellybeans, gummy bears, Fruit Roll-ups™, fruit drinks, snack packs of Oreos, Fig Newtons, Lorna Doones and granola bars.

It's a good idea to leave a couple of these low sugar boxes in strategic locations (one in the classroom, another in the nurse's or principal's office) along with a card that clearly describes the appropriate treatment for your child's hypo. Be sure to replenish the supplies regularly and check that the foods you pack have not passed their "use-by" date.

If your child appears to have low blood sugar episodes at school more often than at home, you may want to test her blood at school to confirm whether she's really hypoglycemic. If she is, her doctor may want to change her insulin dose or reassess her diet to make sure that she's getting enough food.

PREVENTING LATE-MORNING HYPOGLYCEMIA

A common problem for many school children is a delayed recess, which can be as late as 11:00 A.M. Often this gap between breakfast and morning snack is too long, causing hypoglycemia. Some children try to eat during class to prevent hypoglycemia, but this singles them out and may make them feel uncomfortable. Other kids have a small low G.I. snack on their way to school such as dried fruit, flavored milk, a small container of yogurt, whole grain crackers with cheese spread or peanut butter and all-fruit jelly to keep their blood sugar stable.

■

TRY TO INCLUDE A MINIMUM OF ONE LOW G.I. FOOD PER MEAL AND SNACK PER DAY TO ACHIEVE GOOD LONG-TERM DIABETES CONTROL.

■

Chapter 26

TEENAGERS

The teenage years tend to be a time when kids want to challenge the world. And some of these challenges include smoking, drinking, skipping insulin, missing meals and eating whatever! This section provides information that will help parents and teens make good decisions—decisions that will help teens maintain long-term diabetes control and good health.

THE "HOLLOW LEG" SYNDROME

Teenagers tend to grow fast and as a result, are often hungry much of the time. Here's how teens can be more flexible with their diets:

- When they're hungry, teenagers should eat low G.I. foods for maximum fill-up value. Good choices include wholegrain bread, apples, yogurt, pasta, and oatmeal cookies.
- When teens aren't so interested in eating, they can have high G.I. foods in smaller amounts, foods such as white bread, cookies, corn flakes, and rice cakes.

TAKE-OUT FOODS

The problem with take-out foods is that kids usually eat them at irregular times and eat greater amounts of sugary or fatty foods than they should as part of a well-balanced low G.I. diet. Eating additional carbohydrate food will increase blood sugar levels.

But, kids don't have to be different. Incorporating low G.I. foods whenever possible will let teens enjoy take-out foods without compromising their diabetes control; in fact, as long as they keep some pointers in mind, teens can make fairly healthy food choices at take-out restaurants. Hint: Take-out foods that also happen to have low G.I. values include fruit smoothies, ice cream, yogurt, sourdough pretzel nuggets and some types of fresh fruit.

Your kids should also . . .

- choose bottled water, flavored milk or diet decaffeinated soft drinks rather than regular soft drinks.
- combine any high G.I. carbohydrates or saturated fat with low G.I. foods.
- be prepared by having only a light snack after school so they can have an extra snack with their friends.

TYPE OF TAKEOUT FOOD	BEST CHOICES	FOODS TO LIMIT
McDonald's, Burger King, or other hamburger outlets	Chunky chicken salad Small hamburger Chef salad (use low fat or fat-free dressing) Chicken tenders Plain ice cream cone Fruit	Deep-fried food Double meat Extra cheese Fried onion rings French fries Bacon Thick shakes Soft drinks
Pizza takeout/delivery Chinese takeout	Vegetarian topping Simple cheese topping Braised meat or chicken with steamed rice Stirfry vegetables or noodles	Pepperoni Double cheese topping Deep-fried egg or spring rolls or dim sum
Sandwich shops, delis, diners	Whole-grain roll or sandwich bread Veggie burger Grilled chicken salad or pita Milkshakes Frozen yogurt Ice cream or frozen yogurt	Pies Sausage rolls French fries Potato chips
Mexican restaurants such as Taco Bell	Bean burrito Chicken fajita Soft taco Beef taco Tostada with red sauce Frijoles and cheese	Nachos Crispy taco salads Refried beans Guacamole

DRINKING ALCOHOL AND STAYING OUT LATE

Teenagers with diabetes act much like their non-diabetic friends—they may stay out late, sleep in or drink alcohol. They should talk to their doctor, diabetes educator or dietitian for advice on how best to deal with all of these situations.

HOW DOES ALCOHOL AFFECT BLOOD SUGAR LEVELS?

Some drinks, such as beer, mixed drinks, wine coolers and liqueurs, may initially cause elevated blood sugar, or hyperglycemia. But, in general, the biggest problem that comes from combining alcohol with diabetes is actually *low* blood sugar (hypoglycemia), because alcohol prevents the release of stored sugar from the liver. (The body normally calls on these stores if blood sugar levels drop too low.) Unfortunately, since hypoglycemic and excess alcohol symptoms are similar, your teen's hypoglycemia may go undetected. Stress to your teen the importance of *not* drinking alcohol. As an emergency precaution, make sure that someone in your child's group of friends knows that alcohol can cause her blood sugar to drop so that the friend can help you treat the hypoglycemia if it becomes necessary.

FOOD FOR THOUGHT

Your teen should always:
- carry extra food wherever she's going, and
- wear some form of diabetes ID (such as an ID bracelet) in case difficulties arise.

■

TO HELP KEEP BLOOD SUGAR LEVELS STABLE, YOUR TEEN SHOULD BE EDUCATED ON THE DANGERS OF ALCOHOL CONSUMPTION FOR DIABETICS.

■

ALCOHOL AND INSULIN

Drinking on an empty stomach leads to higher blood alcohol levels and, as a result, a greater risk of hypoglycemia. So before your teen goes out for the night, she should inject her insulin and eat a normal-size low G.I. meal—pasta is perfect. She may need to consider lowering her insulin dose, however, if she's lined up lots of activity. She may also need to alter the timing of her doses. (Physical activity tends to lower blood sugar levels.) It would be a good idea for your teen to talk to her diabetes educator to work out an insulin regimen for when she goes out.

WEIGHTY MATTERS

Sometimes the pressures of having a beautiful body seem to clash with the diabetes pressures of eating regularly, eating after exercise and treating low blood sugars.

The good news is, teenagers can maintain a reasonable body weight *and* still control their diabetes.

Becoming overweight is largely an imbalance between activity levels and food intake. If your child honestly thinks she has a weight problem, is worried about how she looks and wants to diet, she should talk to someone about it; the best choices would be a health professional such as her dietitian, doctor or diabetes educator. They can help her plan healthy and effective weight management strategies.

DIETARY DON'TS (THEY *DON'T* WORK!)

No matter how good "quick fix" diets may sound to teenagers, they can all be detrimental to their health. Here are some rules for kids to follow, and the "whys" to back them up:

- Don't eliminate a major food group such as meat, dairy foods or starches in the belief that they're fattening foods. The result is a nutritionally inadequate diet with detrimental long-term consequences.
- Don't try a severe low calorie diet either, because it can dramatically affect your growth and development—and that includes your brain. It's also counterproductive to long-term weight control and will likely bring on a low blood sugar episode.

- Don't reduce, or worse still, skip insulin in an effort to lose weight. This only results in poor diabetes control. Major adjustments to your insulin dose or diet are best made under professional guidance.
- Don't starve yourself or go on eating binges followed by purging. If you find yourself doing this, talk to a health professional about it—you could have an eating disorder.
- Don't be tempted to skip meals or snacks in an attempt to reduce the amount of food that you're eating. Skipping meals and snacks not only upsets diabetes control and causes low blood sugar, but also can leave you feeling very hungry and craving junk foods.

JUGGLING SPORTS COMMITMENTS

Playing sports can provide enormous benefits to diabetes control and feelings of well being. To perform at their best, kids need to monitor the effect that playing a particular sport has on their diabetes control, pay attention to their diet and plan ahead. They should remember to:

- eat extra carbohydrate during periods of strenuous activity
- exercise when levels of insulin are not peaking (although this isn't always practical), and
- inject insulin into an area that is not involved with the vigorous activity.

To deal with before-breakfast training sessions, athletes with diabetes should consume extra low G.I. carbohydrate (such as a bowl of old fashioned oats cooked with milk) before training. After finishing training, they should take their insulin dose, then have a normal breakfast around the usual time.

To cope with training/competition during meal and snack times, athletes should eat carbohydrates appropriate for their activity levels, with some additional carbohydrates to allow for any mealtime delays. A combination of low and high G.I. foods would be best.

When teens know they need additional carbohydrate before competing but have no appetite or desire to eat, they should choose light foods or fluids that sit well in their stomachs, such as fruit smoothies, fruit salads or yogurt.

WORKING PART-TIME

Teens who work part time may need to alter their usual medication and meal routine to fit in with their scheduled work breaks or negotiate adequate breaks with their employer.

Before starting work, teenagers should have a substantial low G.I. meal or snack to help sustain blood sugar levels. It may be a good idea for kids to take extra carbohydrate snacks such as dried fruits, cookies, granola bars and fresh fruit from home so that they can eat them on the run. Sometimes small frequent snacks may need to take the place of a full meal break. If the job is quite busy, teens should make sure that they're prepared with extra high G.I. carbohydrate snacks; she may want to discuss reducing her insulin dose with her doctor.

Chapter 27

THE FOOD PYRAMID FOR ADOLESCENTS AND TEENAGERS

*I*n order to grow and develop properly, an adolescent's diet should follow the food groups of the Food Guide Pyramid that appears on page 00. The recommended caloric level for an adolescent should take into account the child's age, gender, current weight status versus ideal or reasonable body weight*, level of physical activity and growth pattern.

RECOMMENDED FOOD PYRAMID SERVINGS FOR TEENAGERS

As we mentioned earlier, a healthy diet should include low G.I. choices from each of the carbohydrate groups below.

Food group	Servings for teen girls	Servings for teen boys
Bread and cereal	9	11
Vegetable	4	5
Fruit	3	4
Milk	3	3
Meat	2 (total 5 ozs.)	3 (total 8 ozs.)

Discourage your kids from consuming too many caffeine-containing foods, including colas, tea, coffee and chocolate.

DAILY NUTRIENT REQUIREMENTS

Here are some guidelines to help you determine how much your child should be eating.

Calories
Boys
  11–14 years: 41 calories/inch
  15–18 years: 43 calories/inch
Girls
  11–14 years: 36 calories/inch
  15–18 years: 34 calories/inch

Protein
  Approximately 0.4 to 0.5 grams per pound, or 12 to 16 percent of daily calorie intake

Fat
  No more than 30 percent of total calories from fat
  10 percent or less of total fat calories from saturated fat
  Less than 300 milligrams (mg.) of cholesterol

Calcium
1200 to 1500 mg.

Dietary fiber
5 grams plus child's age (Example: A 15-year-old adolescent should get 5 + 15 = 20 grams of fiber each day.)

*Body Mass Index (BMI) categories to identify adolescents at risk of obesity:

Overweight: BMI >30
At risk: BMI = 30

HOW TO CALCULATE BMI:

$$\frac{\text{Your weight (in pounds)} \times 704.5}{\text{Your height (in inches)} \times \text{your height (in inches)}} = \text{Body Mass Index}$$

Example:

$$\frac{100 \text{ pounds} \times 704.5 = 70450}{60 \text{ inches} \times 60 \text{ inches} = 3600 \text{ inches}} = 19.56 \text{ BMI}$$

Discourage your kids from eating too much fat, sodium and sugar. These "empty calorie" foods, quite common in teenagers' diets, can easily squeeze out room for healthier food choices.

Try to include a minimum of one low G.I. food per meal and snack per day to achieve good long-term diabetes control.

Part 5

THE GLYCEMIC INDEX MENU PLANNER FOR CHILDREN AND TEENS

BREAKFAST

LUNCHES AND SANDWICH FILLERS

MAIN MEALS FOR CHILDREN AND TEENS

JUST DESSERTS

LOW G.I. SNACKS

PARTY IDEAS

Chapter 28

BREAKFAST

Breakfast is the meal that starts the day. It's a great opportunity to optimize your use of low G.I. foods because so many breakfast foods—breads, cereals, fresh fruits and dairy foods—are excellent low G.I. food sources. Studies have shown that children who eat a nutritious breakfast will perform better, both physically and mentally, than their hungry peers. A wholesome, nutritious low G.I. breakfast ensures optimal performance until the scheduled morning snack. Just make sure that your kids have enough time to enjoy their breakfast without feeling rushed.

Though breakfast is important, many children don't have large appetites at breakfast time. For small appetites, fruit smoothies and hot chocolate are good starters that will sustain energy levels throughout the morning. Here are some other ideas.

1. **Start with some fruit.**
   Fruit contributes fiber and vitamin C, which helps your body absorb iron.

2. **Try some breakfast cereal.**
   Cereals are important as a source of fiber, vitamin B and iron. When choosing processed breakfast cereals, look for those with a high fiber content (five or more grams per serving). The top four low G.I. cereals for children are: old-fashioned oats, granola, Life, and Special K.

3. **Add milk or yogurt.**
   Fat free or low fat milk can make a valuable contribution to your child's daily calcium intake when you include them at breakfast. Both have low G.I. values, and low fat milk varieties have just as much, or more, calcium as whole milk.

4. **Serve some bread or toast.**
   The lowest G.I. breads are: whole grain pumpernickel (G.I.: 51); sourdough (G.I.: 52); 100% stoneground whole wheat (G.I.: 53); Arnold's sourdough rye (G.I.: 57); and whole wheat pita (G.I.: 57).

FOR TODDLERS

1. Oatmeal and milk and a small glass of apple juice

2. A fruit smoothie—strawberries or peach with milk, yogurt and honey
3. A small yogurt with fresh fruit salad
4. Scrambled eggs on toast with a small cup of milk
5. Graham crackers with peanut butter and all-fruit jelly
6. Cinnamon toast with a cup of milk
7. "Silver dollar" pancakes and milk

FOR SCHOOL CHILDREN

1. French toast, made by lightly soaking thick slices of low G.I. bread in beaten egg and milk. Sprinkle with cinnamon sugar.
2. A bowl of Just Right with sliced canned peaches and low fat milk
3. Sliced strawberries topped with vanilla yogurt and a sprinkle of Bran Buds or granola
4. Peanut butter and all-fruit jelly on low G.I. toast
5. Boiled egg, low G.I. toast and a glass of milk
6. Sourdough English muffin topped with cream cheese

FOR TEENAGERS

1. Bagels
2. Bran, corn or blueberry muffin with all fruit jelly
3. French toast with fresh fruit
4. Fruit smoothie
5. Grilled cheese on wholegrain bread

6. Grilled tomato and cheese on toast/muffins
7. Low G.I. breakfast cereal with milk and fruit
8. Poached eggs on toast
9. Old fashioned oats cooked in low fat milk, topped with sliced peaches or cinnamon applesauce
10. Wholegrain toast with peanut butter, or ham and cheese, or eggs
11. Yogurt and fresh fruit and low fat granola

Chapter 29

LUNCHES AND SANDWICH FILLERS

There's no need for children to regard sandwiches with disdain as long as you keep the fillers tasty and creative. Here are some ideas to get you started.

1. Bacon, lettuce and tomato
2. Egg salad
3. Grilled cheese and tomato
4. Ham, cheese and salsa
5. Hummus and tomato
6. Lean roast beef and light mayonnaise
7. Mozzarella, roasted peppers and arugula
8. Peanut butter and all-fruit jelly
9. Tuna salad
10. Veggie burger

SOME TASTY COMBINATIONS

Looking for some food choices that go particularly well together? Try these combos:

Pita pocket filled with tuna salad, diced tomato and lettuce
Fruit muffin
Small apple and milk
Chicken drumstick with cucumber sticks, cherry tomatoes and rye crackers
Fruit yogurt
Oatmeal cookies

Soft tortilla filled with ham, cheese or turkey with diced tomato, pepper and cucumber
Small container of fresh melon chunks
Frozen flavored milk drink

Roast beef on rye bread with pickle
Container of fruit yogurt
Small container of trail mix

Tossed salad with hard boiled eggs, cheese, olives and chickpeas
Frozen fruit juice
Container of citrus sections

FOOD FOR THOUGHT

- Use different types of bread for variety: Some examples include wholegrain, semolina, sourdough, rye, raisin, muffins, pita, mountain bread, herb bread and soft tortillas.
- Try to make low G.I. sandwiches to help lower the glycemic index for the day.
- Toast sandwiches (such as grilled cheese) the night before; children can eat them cool for lunch the next day for something a little different.

Chapter 30

MAIN MEALS FOR CHILDREN AND TEENS

Once you know where to start, it's easy to make your child's meals interesting and tasty. Here are some ideas to help get the creativity ball rolling.

FOR TODDLERS

1. Grilled cheese on wholegrain toast (cut into triangles) and a sliced apple
2. Light cream cheese and all-fruit jelly on a sourdough English muffin
3. Macaroni and cheese
4. Tomato soup and low G.I. toast

5. Tuna chow mein—canned tuna with fine noodles, stir-fried vegetables, seasoned with soy sauce
6. Vegetable soup with noodles

FOR OLDER CHILDREN AND TEENS

1. Bake a tuna and rice casserole using Uncle Ben's converted or brown rice, peas, corn and strips of red pepper, topped with ½ cup of light cheese sauce made with skim or reduced fat milk.
2. Bake Tex Mex potatoes (sweet potato baked with onion, bacon, taco seasoning, baked beans, grated cheese, sour cream and corn chips).
3. Buy a barbecued chicken, steam corn on the cob and serve with a tossed salad.
4. Buy one or two Chinese take-out stir-fry meals and split them with your family, padding them out with home-cooked low G.I. rice or pasta plus loads of vegetables.
5. Cook a casserole using a good-quality chicken stock and chunks of your child's favorite vegetables, including sweet potato. Serve with brown rice or noodles.
6. Cook spinach and ricotta tortellini, team up with fresh garden vegetables and top with a tomato sauce.
7. Create a one-pot chicken casserole with your favorite vegetables and chunks of baby new potatoes.
8. Enjoy a risotto made with a low G.I. rice, lean meat, fish or chicken and a variety of vegetables.
9. Grill a steak and serve with a trio of low G.I. vegetables—sweet potato, corn and peas.

10. Grill or barbecue steak (or chicken or fish) and serve with a variety of low G.I. vegetables (sweet potato, corn and peas) and crusty whole grain rolls.
11. Make a lasagna—beef and cheese or vegetarian—and serve it with a crispy green salad with lettuce and celery and colorful pepper strips.
12. Serve chili beans and beef with a soft tortilla bread or tacos and a salad.
13. Serve grilled or barbecued sausages and mashed potatoes made with a 50–50 mixture of new potato and sweet potato and served with corn on the cob.
14. Serve your favorite pasta (al dente) with a meat sauce or vegetable salsa, and couple it with lightly steamed green vegetables.
15. Stir-fry beef, chicken or fish and serve with Basmati rice or noodles.
16. Stir-fry chicken, meat or fish with mixed green vegetables. Serve with brown rice or Chinese noodles.
17. Team spaghetti bolognese with a green salad.
18. Try a corn and green pea frittata, made with eggs and fresh vegetables or a can of corn and a small packet of frozen peas.
19. Wrap a fish fillet dressed with herbs and lemon, or tomato and onion, in foil and bake. Serve with a heavy grain bread roll and salad.

OTHER MEAL IDEAS

1. Make vegetable parcels by combining chopped cooked broccoli, grated carrot, chopped shallots and sweet corn with ricotta cheese and grated cheddar. Wrap in phyllo pastry and bake until golden.
2. Scoop commercial pasta sauce on pasta with a sprinkle of Parmesan cheese. Add mushrooms, peppers and other vegetables to the sauce to boost the nutrient value.
3. Serve a casserole with chunky vegetables and sweet potato cubes served with Basmati rice or elbow macaroni.
4. Thread cubes of chicken, beef or fish onto skewers with button mushrooms, onions and peppers for a kebab.
5. Microwave a potato and top with broccoli and cheddar cheese.
6. Microwave a veggie burger.
7. Serve nachos or tacos with beef and bean topping, avocado, shredded lettuce, tomato, and reduced-fat grated cheddar cheese.
8. Savor a lentil or split pea soup.

Chapter 31

JUST DESSERTS

Children love desserts, which can add calcium and vitamin C to their meals if they're based on low fat dairy foods and fruits. Recipes incorporating fruit for sweetness will have more fiber and lower G.I. values than recipes with sugar. What's more, desserts are usually carbohydrate rich, which means they help children feel more full, and reduce the tendency for late night nibbles.

If you don't have time to prepare a dessert, try serving a bowl of in-season fruit or a fruit platter with cheese or yogurt. Remember, temperate climate fruits such as apples, pears, peaches, citrus and berries tend to have the lowest G.I. values.

For any of the following suggestions, you should

substitute whole milk or whole milk products for children under two years old unless otherwise advised.

QUICK AND EASY LOW G.I. DESSERTS

Most everyone looks forward to a sweet, tasty dessert to top off a meal. Here are some simple ideas to end your child's meal in grand style.

1. Combine low fat ice cream and strawberries.
2. Bake apples whole, and stuff them with dried fruit or tapioca pudding.
3. Enjoy a fruit salad topped with low fat yogurt.
4. Make a fruit crisp: Top cooked fruit with a crumble mixture of oats, a little melted margarine (poly- or monounsaturated) and honey.
5. Slice a firm banana into some low fat custard.
6. Top canned fruit (peaches or pears) with low fat ice cream, low fat custard or pudding.
7. Wrap sliced apple, raisins, nuts and cinnamon in a sheet of phyllo pastry (brushed with milk, not fat) and bake as a strudel.
8. Make a winter fruit salad with segments of citrus fruits and raisins soaked in orange juice and honey.
9. Stew peaches or nectarines and serve them with low fat frozen yogurt.
10. Make a pudding cooked in low fat milk.
11. Enjoy a small dish of frozen yogurt.

Chapter 32

LOW G.I. SNACKS

Low G.I. foods, as part of your children's meals and snacks, not only help to prevent low blood sugar, but also provide the long-term energy your young ones need to make it through a busy day. Consider these tasty choices.

FOR TODDLERS

1. Blueberry or applesauce muffin
2. Cup of milk and an oatmeal cookie
3. Frozen yogurt
4. Fruit yogurt
5. Raisin toast spread lightly with low fat cream cheese

CHILDREN WITH TYPE 1 DIABETES

6. Slice of fresh low G.I. bread with margarine and all-fruit jelly
7. Sliced apple
8. Small bowl of dried fruit—apricot halves, dried apples and berries

FOR SCHOOL-AGE CHILDREN

1. Canned fruit snack pack
2. Carrot, celery and zucchini sticks with peanut butter dip
3. Cheese melted on low G.I. toast
4. Frozen yogurt on a stick
5. Granola bar
6. Fruit plate of sliced apple, orange rings, grapes or melon chunks
7. Ice cream cone
8. Tangerines or a bunch of grapes
9. Mini corn cob
10. Corn muffin
11. Vegetable soup with a crusty wholegrain roll
12. Yogurt with Grape-Nuts or low fat granola

FOR TEENAGERS

1. Apple or pear
2. Muffins or raisin bread
3. Leftovers—pizza, rice, noodles
4. Low fat ice cream
5. Low fat milk
6. Nachos—corn chips and melted cheese
7. Nutri-Grain bars
8. Pasta snack
9. Smoothie
10. Grilled sandwich made with low G.I. bread

Chapter 33

PARTY IDEAS

Your child shouldn't miss out on party fun and fare just because she has diabetes. Within reason, relax her diet for that special meal or snack and allow a moderate number of party treats. Having one slice of birthday cake is sensible, for example, but going back for a third helping is not. Encourage her to bring home the goodie bag, which she can have either as dessert that evening or before exercise later. An occasional rise in blood sugar level on special occasions does no harm. It's what you do the remainder of the time that is more important.

On the day of the party, keep the insulin dose the same (even though it is likely that she'll eat extra). Remember that she may be more active at the party, which would allow her to eat the extra party food without increasing her blood sugar levels too dramatically.

If her blood sugar is high after the party, don't panic. Make sure she eats her dinner and bedtime snack so that her blood sugar levels don't drop rapidly overnight.

■

MANY PARENTS ARE SURPRISED AT HOW GOOD THEIR CHILD'S BLOOD SUGAR READINGS ARE AFTER PARTIES.

■

PARTY FARE

When children go to parties, what they eat depends largely on what the hosts offer. If you know the party hosts, you can call them ahead of time to find out what they're serving. If that's not an option for you, you could have your child bring a tasty treat for all the guests to share.

Here are some ideas of foods you could bring, or serve when the party is at your house:

> Cakes, cookies, ice cream (made with artificial sweeteners, alternative sweeteners such as fructose, fruit juice, or fruit purees, or reduced amounts of sugar)
> Calzones
> Chicken nuggets
> Chili
> Chips and salsa
> Decaf diet beverages

Lasagna
Nuts
Sloppy Joe pitas
Spaghetti and meatballs
Sweet potato fries
Tacos
Tortilla wraps
Veggies and dips
White pizza

Part 6

YOUR QUESTIONS ANSWERED

THE MEAL SKIPPERS

NO SPECIAL TREATS REQUIRED

CANDY CONCERNS

HYPOGLYCEMIA AFTER SPORTS

INFANT AND TODDLER CONCERNS

Chapter 34

THE MEAL SKIPPERS

My daughter refuses to eat breakfast before going to school and I'm worried that she will become hypoglycemic on the way to school. What should I do?

Breakfast is an important meal to start the day and skipping this meal should not be an option for any child with diabetes. Breakfast provides you with a great opportunity to include plenty of low G.I. foods because many breakfast items—breads, cereals, fresh fruits and dairy foods—have low G.I. values. Some children don't have large appetites at breakfast time, so it is important to optimize carbohydrate intake.

Make sure there is plenty of time to enjoy a good breakfast. Milkshakes, fruit smoothies and hot chocolate are good starters. All of these foods have low G.I. values that will sustain blood sugar levels for longer periods. And negotiate foods that she will eat—they needn't necessarily be traditional breakfast foods. Check the low G.I. breakfast list on page 95 for some creative ideas.

She may prefer two small low G.I. snacks (one at breakfast and one on the way to school), which will ensure that she gets enough carbohydrate to minimize the risk of low blood sugar.

When my son is invited to parties he gets so busy playing that he hardly eats and always ends up hypoglycemic. What should I do?

Give your son a low G.I. snack before he goes to the party so that what he eats once he gets there will not be as important. Low G.I. snacks will help him maintain blood sugar control and will lessen the blood sugar effects of any party foods he does eat.

My son eats too much after school, then has high blood sugar readings and is never hungry at dinnertime. What should I do?

Your son is hungry and eating large quantities of food in the afternoon when the effects of his long-acting insulin are wearing off; that's why his blood sugar level is elevated.

First, watch the foods he eats for his afternoon snack. High fat snack foods, such as chips or sweet cookies, don't satisfy an appetite. Try combining these foods with some low G.I. choices (such as fruit, sandwiches made with wholegrain breads or rolls, or milk) that will satisfy his appetite and have a minimal impact on his blood sugar.

Try to understand why he's so hungry. Is he eating enough during the day? Providing low G.I. food choices for him to eat throughout the day, particularly his school lunch, may help alleviate that ravenous after-school appetite.

Is he eating because he's bored? Suggest that once he's had his snack he get away from food and get busy.

Alternatively, maybe his insulin regime can be adjusted. He might try dividing his pre-dinner insulin dose into two separate injections by giving himself the short-acting insulin after school. That way he'll have adequate insulin to cope with his large after-school appetite. He may then take his long-acting insulin before supper. Effectively, he'll be giving himself three injections of insulin per day so that the peak action of insulin is better matched to his food intake and blood sugar profile. Discuss these options with your son's diabetes care team.

NO SPECIAL TREATS REQUIRED

I spend weekends baking special sugar-free cakes and cookies for my son's school lunch to try to give him more variety, but these foods always come home uneaten. Can you suggest any special recipe books?

There's no need to use special sugar-free recipes or artificial sweeteners: Using moderate amounts of sugar in cooking is fine and won't interfere with your son's diabetes control as long as you count these foods as part of his total carbohydrate intake. Bake your family's favorite recipes, and remember that it's more likely that you'll need to reduce the fat content of your recipes than the sugar content.

CANDY CONCERNS

My child is very active during playtime at school so I pack candy in his lunch box every day to prevent low blood sugar. Now he eats more candy than he ever did before he was diagnosed with diabetes. Does this seem right?

Your child should not need candy every day to prevent dips in blood sugar. Even if he is very active at play, his regular insulin dose and food intake should be appropriate for his activity level. Additional carbohydrate foods are only required for extra strenuous activity. If you find that your child needs to eat extra food regularly, discuss his current insulin regimen with his doctor and have a registered dietitian review his calorie intake.

HYPOGLYCEMIA AFTER SPORTS

My son is very active and attends track practice three afternoons a week. He always eats extra foods before training but seems to experience hypoglycemia in the late evening after each session. Is there something more he should be doing?

Delayed hypoglycemia after strenuous activity is usually an indication that your son requires either more carbohydrate or less insulin. During the activity he may have used the glucose stored in his liver, and it isn't until later in the evening, when his body tries to replenish its stores, that the hypoglycemia occurs. He can prevent this from happening by eating some high G.I. carbohydrate prior to, during or immediately after the event. Alternatively, he could reduce his insulin dose if he doesn't want to eat more carbohydrate. He should make sure that his dinner and bedtime snack contain additional low G.I. carbohydrate foods to sustain his blood sugar levels overnight.

Appetite is often a good guide to help determine whether your son needs additional carbohydrate. We recommend that he eat extra low G.I. foods at dinner and/or bedtime to match his appetite after very strenuous activities. It may be a good idea for your son to check his blood sugar levels more frequently—at least temporarily—before, during, immediately following and approximately four to six hours after his training sessions. The results will provide him with valuable blood sugar information so that he can make better decisions regarding any insulin/food changes.

INFANT AND TODDLER CONCERNS

How can I tell if my breastfed baby is getting enough breast milk to avoid hypoglycemia?

If your baby is thriving, gaining the appropriate amount of weight, has an adequate number of wet diapers, appears settled after feedings and is demand feeding every two to three hours throughout the day, the chances are that your baby is receiving enough and doing well. You can also regularly monitor her blood sugar level to reassure yourself that you're meeting her needs.

Should I introduce solids to my baby before she's five months old?

No. There is no benefit in introducing solids before five months of age. A baby's digestive system is still immature and not ready to cope with solid foods before then. Introducing foods earlier may increase your baby's chances of developing food allergies and diarrhea (due to undigested food); it can also lead to poor growth. If you think your baby is hungry, offer more breast milk or formula feedings until she's ready to start solids.

What is the best way to manage low blood sugars in an infant?

Treat hypoglycemia by giving your infant glucose syrup either from a plastic eye dropper or a soft plastic spoon, followed by a breast- or formula feeding as soon as possible.

My toddler is so tired by the end of the day, he won't eat his evening meal and I am frightened that his blood sugar will drop in the middle of the night. What should I do?

It isn't unusual for tired toddlers to be uninterested in the evening meal; in fact, they can often be quite distracted if the whole family is sitting down together. Feeding your toddler earlier in the evening (5:00 or 5:30 P.M.) before fatigue sets in may help. Then they can sit with the family at the later mealtime without the pressure. If they consume more food during your family's evening meal, it's a bonus.

Another approach would be to give toddlers their main meal at lunchtime when their appetites may be better. You can then offer a lighter evening meal, such as sandwiches, fruit or yogurt. Check the meal and snack suggestions on pages 102 and 108 for ways to incorporate low G.I. foods into your child's usual food choices. A bottle or cup of milk before bed is a common routine in this age group and may help to satisfy their appetite for a longer period since low G.I. foods (such as milk) make them feel fuller longer. It also can be helpful and reassuring to monitor your child's blood sugar at bedtime.

My two-year-old girl's blood sugars are never stable. How can I determine what I'm doing wrong?

Be reassured that you are not the only parent of a toddler with diabetes who is frustrated with unstable diabetes control. We don't aim for tight control because detecting and treating low blood sugar in this age group is a difficult task, because toddlers are too young to recognize the symptoms. Experts accept a wider blood sugar range in this age group because kids' activity levels are erratic and their food intake can be unpredictable. Your child's HbA1c results are often a better indication of their overall diabetes control than the highly fluctuating daily blood tests. (Hemoglobin A1c is a blood test that gives a person's blood sugar average for the prior two to three months.)

Incorporating low G.I. foods over the course of the day may help to minimize the rapid blood sugar fluctuations, but it certainly won't prevent them. If you can manage your toddler's diabetes so that she is free of hypoglycemia and ketones, you're doing a fabulous job.

My two-year-old son is about to start childcare. How can I be sure that his diabetes will be managed properly?

One of the hardest things about being a parent is letting go as your toddler becomes more independent and others assume responsibility for his well being. You need to feel confident that the staff is able to manage his diabetes: They need to be made aware of his usual routines and know how to recognize and treat symptoms of hypoglycemia.

In our experience, there have been no difficulties with children attending childcare: The days are structured and the meals they supply are nutritious and appropriate. If you feel that this isn't the case, though, you could send your child's food with him each day. Your diabetes educator may be able to visit the center or provide you with written information to pass on to the staff.

Part 7

THE G.I. TABLES

HOW TO USE THE G.I. TABLES

THE GLYCEMIC INDEX TABLES

Chapter 35

HOW TO USE THE G.I. TABLES

The following table is an A to Z listing of the glycemic index values of commonly eaten foods in the United States and Canada. Approximately 350 different foods are listed, including some new values for foods tested only recently.

The glycemic index shown next to each food is the average for that food using glucose as the standard (i.e., glucose has a glycemic index of 100, with other foods rated accordingly). The average may represent the mean of 10 studies of that food worldwide or only two to four studies. In a few instances, American data is different from the rest of the world and we show that data rather than the average. Rice and oatmeal fall into this category.

To check on a food's glycemic index, simply look

for it by name in the alphabetic list. You may also find it under a food type (e.g., fruit, cookies).

We've included in the tables the carbohydrate (CHO) and fat content of a sample serving of the food to help you and your child keep track of the amount of fat and carbohydrate in her diet. The sample serving is not the recommended serving—it is just an example of a serving. The glycemic index does not depend on serving size because it is a ranking of the glycemic effect of foods using carbohydrate-equivalent portion sizes. Children can eat more of a low G.I. food or less of a high G.I. food and achieve the same blood sugar levels.

Remember that when you're choosing foods for your family, the glycemic index isn't the only thing to consider: As far as blood sugar levels are concerned, you should also consider the amount of carbohydrate they're eating, and the fat, fiber and micronutrient content of their diet is also important. A dietitian can guide you further with good food choices for your children; see "For More Information" on page 143 for advice on finding a dietitian.

Chapter 35

THE GLYCEMIC INDEX TABLES

The G.I. values in these tables are correct at the time of publication. However, the formulation of some commercial foods can change, which can alter the glycemic index. Check our web page for revised and new data:
www.biochem.usyd.edu.au/~jennie/GI/glycemic_index.html

Note: You'll notice that certain foods have G.I. values exceeding 100. When measuring the glycemic index, experts use bread and glucose as the two reference foods, the standards against which the glycemic values of all other foods are measured. Glucose is used because it is the end product of digestion, and white bread is used because it is a staple in many of our diets. But foods with higher G.I. values do exist.

A–Z OF FOODS WITH GLYCEMIC INDEX, CARBOHYDRATE, AND FAT

Food	Glycemic Index	Fat (g per svg.)	CHO (g per svg.)
Agave nectar (90% fructose syrup), 1 tablespoon	11	0	12
All-Bran™, Kellogg's, breakfast cereal, ½ cup, 1 oz.	42 (av)	1	22
All-Bran with Extra Fiber™, Kellogg's, breakfast cereal, ½ cup, 1 oz.	51 (av)	1	20
Angel food cake, 1/12 cake, 1 oz.	67	trace	17
Apple, 1 medium, 5 ozs.	38 (av)	0	18
Apple, dried, 1 oz.	29	0	24
Apple juice, unsweetened, 1 cup, 8 ozs.	40	0	29
Apple cinnamon muffin, from mix, 1 muffin,	44	5	26
Apricots, fresh, 3 medium, 3 ozs.	57	0	12
canned, light syrup, 3 halves	64	0	14
dried, 5 halves	31	0	13
Apricot jam, no added sugar, 1 tablespoon	55	0	17
Apricot and honey muffin, low fat, from mix, 1 muffin	60	4	27
Arborio risotto rice, white, boiled, ⅔ cup	69	0	35
Bagel, 1 small, plain, 2 ozs.	72	1	38
Baked beans, ½ cup, 4 ozs.	48 (av)	1	24
Banana bread, 1 slice, 3 ozs.	47	7	46
Banana, raw, 1 medium, 5 ozs.	55 (av)	0	32
Banana, oat and honey muffin, low fat from mix, 1 muffin, small	65	4	28
Barley, pearled, boiled, ½ cup, 2.6 ozs.	25 (av)	0	22
Basmati white rice, boiled, 1 cup, 6 ozs.	58	0	50
Beans and legumes			
Baked beans, ½ cup, 4 ozs.	48 (av)	1	24
Black beans, boiled, ¾ cup, 4.3 ozs.	30	1	21
Black bean soup, ½ cup, 4½ ozs.	64	2	19
Blackeyed peas, canned, ½ cup, 4 ozs.	42	1	16
Broad beans, canned, ½ cup	79	1	9
Butter beans, boiled, ½ cup, 4 ozs.	31 (av)	0	16
Cannellini beans	31	0	16
Chickpeas (garbanzo beans), canned, drained, ½ cup, 4 ozs.	42	2	15
boiled, ½ cup, 3 ozs.	33 (av)	2	23

Food	Glycemic Index	Fat (g per svg.)	CHO (g per svg.)
Fava beans, frozen, boiled, ½ cup, 3 ozs.	79	0	17
Green pea soup, canned, ready to serve, 1 cup, 9 ozs.	66	3	27
Kidney beans, red, boiled, ½ cup, 3 ozs.	27 (av)	0	20
Kidney beans, red, canned and drained, ½ cup, 4.3 ozs.	52	0	19
Lentils, green and brown, boiled, ½ cup, 3 ozs.	30 (av)	0	16
Lentils, red, boiled, 1.4 cup, 4 ozs.	26 (av)	0	27
Lentil soup, Unico, canned, 1 cup, 8 ozs.	44	1	24
Lima beans, baby, frozen, ½ cup, 3 ozs.	32	0	17
Mung beans, boiled, ½ cup, 3½ ozs.	38	1	18
Navy beans, boiled, ½ cup, 3 ozs.	38 (av)	0	19
Pea soup, split with ham, canned, 1 cup, 5 ½ ozs.	66	3	25
Peas, green, fresh, frozen, boiled, ½ cup, 2.7 ozs.	48 (av)	0	11
Peas dried, boiled, ½ cup, 2 ozs.	22	0	7
Pinto beans, canned, ½ cup, 4 ozs.	45	1	18
Pinto beans, soaked, boiled, ½ cup, 3 ozs.	39	0	22
Soy beans, boiled, ½ cup, 3 ozs.	18 (av)	7	10
Split peas, yellow, boiled, ½ cup, 3 ½ ozs.	32	0	21
Beets, canned, drained, ½ cup, 3 ozs.	64	0	5
Black bean soup, ½ cup, 4 ½ ozs.	64	2	19
Black beans, boiled, ¾ cup, 4.3 ozs.	30	1	21
Black bread, dark rye, 1 slice, 1.7 ozs.	76	1	18
Blackeyed peas, canned, ½ cup, 4 ozs.	42	1	16
Blueberry muffin, 1 muffin, 2 ozs.	59	4	27
Bran			
All-Bran with Extra Fiber™, Kellogg's, ½ cup, 1 oz	51	1	20
Bran Buds™, Kellogg's, ⅓ cup	58	1	14
Bran Flakes, Post, ⅔ cup, 1 oz.	74	1	22
Multi-Bran Chex™, General Mills, 1 cup, 2. ozs.	58	1.5	49
Oat bran, 1 tablespoon	55	1	7
Oat bran muffin, 2 ozs.	60	4	28
Rice bran, extruded, 1 tablespoon	19	2	3
Bran muffin, 1	60	8	34
Breads			
Dark rye, Black bread, 1 slice, 1.7 ozs.	76	1	18
Dark rye, Schinkenbröt, 1 slice, 2 ozs.	86	1	22
French baguette, 1 oz.	95	1	15

Food	Glycemic Index	Fat (g per svg.)	CHO (g per svg.)
Gluten-free bread, 1 slice, 1 oz.	90	1	18
Hamburger bun, 1 prepacked bun, 1½ ozs.	61	2	22
Kaiser roll, 1, 2 ozs.	73	2	34
Light deli (American) rye, 1 slice, 1 oz.	68	1	16
Melba toast, 6 pieces, 1 oz.	70	2	23
Pita bread, whole wheat, 6½ inch loaf, 2 ozs.	57	2	35
Pumpernickel, whole grain, 1 slice, 1 oz.	51	1	16
Rye bread, 1 slice, 1 oz.	65	1	15
Sourdough, 1 slice, 1½ ozs.	52	1	20
Natural Ovens 100% Whole Grain, 1 slice, 1.2 ozs.	51	0	17
Natural Ovens Hunger Filler, 1 slice, 1.2 ozs.	59	0	16
Natural Ovens Natural Wheat, 1 slice, 1.2 ozs.	59	0	16
Natural Ovens Happiness, 1 slice, 1.1 ozs.	63	0	15
Sourdough rye, Arnold's, 1 slice, 1½ ozs.	57	1	21
White, 1 slice, 1 oz.	70 (av)	1	12
100% stoneground whole wheat, 1 slice, 1½ ozs.	53	1	12
Whole wheat, 1 slice, 1 oz.	69 (av)	1	13
Bread stuffing from mix, 2 ozs.	74	5	13
Breakfast cereals			
All-Bran™, Kellogg's, breakfast cereal, ½ cup, 1 oz.	42 (av)	1	22
All-Bran with Extra Fiber™, Kellogg's, ½ cup, 1 oz.	51	1	20
Bran Buds™, Kellogg's, ⅓ cup	58	1	14
Bran Flakes, Post, ⅔ cup, 1 oz.	74	1	22
Cheerios™, General Mills, 1 cup, 1 oz.	74	2	23
Cocoa Krispies™, Kellogg's, 1 cup, 1 oz.	77	1	27
Corn Bran™, Quaker Crunchy, ¾ cup, 1 oz.	75	1	23
Corn Chex™, Nabisco, 1 cup, 1 oz.	83	0	26
Corn Flakes™, Kellogg's, 1 cup, 1 oz.	84 (av)	0	24
Corn Pops™, 1 cup	80	0	27
Cream of Wheat, instant, 1 packet, 1 oz.	74	0	21
Cream of Wheat, old fashioned, ¾ cup, cooked, 6 ozs.	66	0	21
Crispix™, Kellogg's, 1 cup, 1 oz.	87	0	25
Frosted Flakes™, Kellogg's, ¾ cup, 1 oz.	55	0	28
Golden Grahams™, General Mills, ¾ cup, 1.6 ozs.	71	1	25
Grapenuts™, Post, ½ cup, 1 oz.	71	1	47
Grapenuts Flakes™, Post, ¾ cup, 1 oz.	80	1	24
Just Right™, ¾ cup	60	1	36

Food	Glycemic Index	Fat (g per svg.)	CHO (g per svg.)
Life™, Quaker, ¾ cup, 1 oz.	66	1	25
Mini Wheats (whole wheat), 1 cup	58	0	21
Muesli, natural muesli, ⅔ cup, 1½ ozs.	56	3	28
Muesli, breakfast cereal, toasted, ⅔ cup, 2 ozs.	43	3	41
Multi-Bran Chex™, General Mills, 1 cup, 2 ozs.	58	1.5	49
Nutri-grain™ breakfast cereal, 1 cup	66	0	20
Oat bran, raw, 1 tablespoon	55	1	7
Oat bran™, Quaker Oats, breakfast cereal, ¾ cup, 1 oz.	50	1	23
Oatmeal (made with water), old fashioned, cooked, ½ cup, 4 ozs.	49 (av)	1	12
Oats, 1-minute, Quaker Oats, 1 cup, cooked	66	2	25
Puffed Wheat™, Quaker, 2 cups, 1 oz.	80	0	22
Raisin Bran™, Kellogg's, ¾ cup, 1 oz.	73	0	32
Rice bran, 1 tablespoon	19	2	5
Rice Chex™, General Mills, 1¼ cups, 1 oz.	89	0	27
Rice Krispies™, Kellogg's, 1¼ cups, 1 oz.	82	0	26
Shredded Wheat™, Post, breakfast cereal, ½ cup, 1 oz.	83	1	23
Shredded wheat, 1 biscuit, ⅘ oz.	62	0	19
Shredded wheat, spoonsize, ⅔ cup, 1.2 ozs.	58	0	27
Smacks™, Kellogg's, ¾ cup, 1 oz.	56	1	27
Special K™, Kellogg's, 1 cup, 1 oz.	54	0	22
Team Flakes™, Nabisco, ¾ cup, 1 oz.	82	0	25
Total™, General Mills, ¾ cup, 1 oz.	76	1	24
WeetaBix™, 2 biscuits, 1.2 ozs.	75	1	28
Breton wheat crackers, 6	67	6	14
Broad beans, canned, ½ cup	79	1	9
Buckwheat groats, cooked, ½ cup, 2.7 ozs.	54 (av)	1	20
Bulgur, cooked, ⅔ cup, 4 ozs.	48 (av)	0	23
Bun, hamburger, 1 prepacked bun, 1.7 ozs.	61	2	22
Butter beans, boiled, ½ cup, 4 ozs.	31 (av)	0	16
Cakes			
Angel food cake, 1 slice, 1/12 cake, 1 oz.	67	trace	17
Banana bread, 1 slice, 3 ozs.	47	7	46
Chocolate fudge cake, pkt. mix, with dark Dutch fudge frosting, Betty Crocker, 1/12 of cake, with 2 tablespoons frosting	38	17	54
French vanilla cake, pkt. mix, with vanilla frosting, Betty Crocker, 1/12 of cake, with 2 tablespoons frosting	42	15	58

Food	Glycemic Index	Fat (g per svg.)	CHO (g per svg.)
Pound cake, homemade, 1 slice, 3 ozs.	54	15	42
Sponge cake, 1 slice, 1/12 cake, 2 ozs.	46	4	32
Capellini pasta, cooked, 1 cup, 6 ozs.	45	1	53
Cannellini beans, boiled, 1/2 cup, 4 ozs.	31	0	16
Cantaloupe, raw, 1/4 small, 6 1/2 ozs.	65	0	16
Carrots, peeled, boiled, 1/2 cup, 2.4 ozs.	49	0	3
Cereal grains			
Barley, pearled, boiled, 1/2 cup, 2.6 ozs.	25 (av)	0	22
Bulgur, cooked, 1/2 cup, 3 ozs.	48 (av)	0	17
Couscous, cooked, 1/2 cup, 3 ozs.	65 (av)	0	21
Corn			
Cornmeal, whole grain, from mix, cooked, 1/3 cup, 1.4 ozs.	68	1	30
Corn, canned, drained, 1/2 cup, 3 ozs.	55 (av)	1	15
Taco shells, 2 shells, 1 oz.	68	5	17
Rice			
Basmati, white, boiled, 1 cup, 6 ozs.	58	0	50
Brown, 1 cup, 6 ozs.	55 (av)	0	37
Converted™, Uncle Ben's, 1 cup, 6 ozs.	44	38	
Instant, cooked, 1 cup, 6 ozs.	87	0	37
Long grain, white, 1 cup, 6 ozs.	56 (av)	0	42
Parboiled, 1 cup, 6 ozs.	48	0	38
Rice cakes, plain, 3 cakes, 1 oz.	82	1	23
Short grain, white, 1 cup, 6 ozs.	72	0	42
Chana dal, 1/2 cup, 4 ozs.	8	3	28
Cheerios™, General Mills, breakfast cereal, 1 cup, 1 oz.	74	2	23
Cherries, 10 large cherries, 3 ozs.	22	0	10
Chickpeas (garbanzo beans),			
canned, drained, 1/2 cup, 4 ozs.	42	2	15
boiled, 1/2 cup, 3 ozs.	33 (av)	2	23
Chocolate butterscotch muffin, low fat from mix, 1 muffin	53	4	28
Chocolate, bar, 1 1/2 ozs.	49	14	26
Chocolate Flavor, Nestle Quik™ (made with water), 3 teaspoons	53	0	14
Chocolate fudge cake, pkt. mix, with dark Dutch fudge frosting, Betty Crocker, 1/12 of cake, with 2 tablespoons frosting	38	17	54
Coca-Cola™, soft drink, 1 can	63	0	41
Cocoa Krispies™, Kellogg's, breakfast cereal, 1 cup, 1 oz.	77	1	27

Food	Glycemic Index	Fat (g per svg.)	CHO (g per svg.)
Corn			
Cornmeal (polenta), 1/3 cup, 1.4 ozs.	68	1	30
Corn, canned and drained, 1/2 cup, 3 ozs.	55 (av)	1	15
Corn Bran™, Quaker Crunchy, breakfast cereal, 3/4 cup, 1 oz.	75	1	23
Corn Chex™, General Mills, breakfast cereal, 1 cup, 1 oz.	83	0	
Corn chips, 1 oz.	72	10	16
Corn Flakes™, Kellogg's, breakfast cereal, 1 cup, 1 oz.	84 (av)	0	24
Corn Pops™, 1 cup	80	0	27
Cornmeal, from mix, cooked, 1/3 cup, 1.4 ozs.	68	1	30
Cookies			
Graham crackers, 4 squares, 1 oz.	74	3	22
Milk Arrowroot, 3 cookies, 1/2 oz.	69	2	9
Oatmeal, 1 cookie, 2/3 oz.	55	3	12
Shortbread, 4 small cookies, 1 oz.	64	7	19
Social Tea™ biscuits, Nabisco, 4 cookies, 2/3 oz.	55	3	13
Vanilla wafers, 7 cookies, 1 oz.	77	4	21
see also Crackers			
Couscous, cooked, 2/3 cup, 4 ozs.	65 (av)	0	21
Crackers			
Breton wheat crackers, 6	67	6	14
Crispbread, 3 crackers, 2/3 oz.	81	0	15
Kavli™ All Natural Whole Grain Crispbread, 4 wafers, 1 oz.	71	1	16
Premium saltine crackers, 8 crackers, 1 oz.	74	3	17
Rice cakes, plain, 3 cakes, 1 oz.	82	1	23
Ryvita™ Tasty Dark Rye Whole Grain Crisp Bread, 2 slices, 2/3 oz.	69	1	16
Stoned wheat thins, 3 crackers, 4/5 oz.	67	2	15
Water cracker, Carr's, 3 king size crackers, 4/5 oz.	78	2	18
Cranberry juice cocktail, 8 ozs.	52	0	31
Cream of Wheat, instant, 1 packet, 1 oz.	74	0	21
Cream of Wheat, old fashioned, 3/4 cup, cooked, 6 ozs.	66	0	21
Crispix™, Kellogg's, breakfast cereal, 1 cup, 1 oz.	87	0	25
Croissant, medium, 1.2 ozs.	67	14	27
Cupcake, with icing and cream filling, 1 cake	73	3	26
Custard, 3/4 cup, 4.4 ozs.	43	5	36
Dairy foods and nondairy substitutes			
Ice cream, 10% fat, vanilla, 1/2 cup, 2.2 ozs.	61 (av)	7	16

Food	Glycemic Index	Fat (g per svg.)	CHO (g per svg.)
Ice milk, vanilla, ½ cup, 2.2 ozs.	50	3	15
Milk, whole, 1 cup, 8 ozs.	27 (av)	9	11
skim, 1 cup, 8 ozs.	32	0	12
chocolate flavored, 1%, 1 cup, 8 ozs.	34	3	26
Pudding, ½ cup, 4.4 ozs.	43	4	27
Soy milk, 1 cup, 8 ozs.	31	7	14
Tofu frozen dessert (nondairy), low fat, ½ cup, 2 ozs.	115	1	21
Yogurt			
nonfat, fruit flavored, with sugar, 8 ozs.	33	0	30
nonfat, plain, artificial sweetener, 8 ozs.	14	0	17
nonfat, fruit flavored, artificial sweetener, 8 ozs.	14	0	17
Dates, dried, 5, 1.4 ozs.	103	0	27
Doughnut with cinnamon and sugar, 1.6 ozs.	76	11	29
Fanta™, soft drink, 1 can	68	0	47
Fava beans, frozen, boiled, ½ cup, 3 ozs.	79	0	17
Fettucine, cooked, 1 cup, 6 ozs.	32	1	57
Fish sticks, frozen, oven-cooked, fingers, 3½ sticks	38	14	24
Flan (creme caramel), ½ cup, 4 ozs.	65	5	23
French baguette bread, 1 oz., about one 1-inch slice	95	0	15
French fries, large, 4.3 ozs.	75	22	46
French vanilla cake, pkt. mix, with vanilla frosting, Betty Crocker, 1/12 of cake, with 2 tablespoons frosting	42	15	58
Frosted Flakes™, Kellogg's, breakfast cereal, ¾ cup, 1 oz.	55	0	28
Fructose, pure, 3 packets	23 (av)	0	10
Fruit cocktail, canned in natural juice, ½ cup, 4 ozs.	55	0	15
Fruits and fruit products			
Agave nectar (90% fructose syrup), 1 tablespoon	11	0	12
Apple, 1 medium, 5 ozs.	38 (av)	0	18
Apple, dried, 1 oz.	29	0	24
Apple juice, unsweetened, 1 cup, 8 ozs.	40	0	29
Apricots, fresh, 3 medium, 3.3 ozs.	57	0	12
canned, light syrup, 3 halves	64	0	19
dried, 1 oz.	31	0	13
Apricot jam, no added sugar, 1 tablespoon	55	0	17
Banana, raw, 1 medium, 5 ozs.	55 (av)	0	32
Cherries, 10 large, 3 ozs.	22	0	10
Cranberry juice cocktail, 8 ozs.	52	0	31

CHILDREN WITH TYPE 1 DIABETES

Food	Glycemic Index	Fat (g per svg.)	CHO (g per svg.)
Dates, dried, 5, 1.4 ozs.	103	0	27
Fruit cocktail, canned in natural juice, ½ cup, 4 ozs.	55	0	15
Grapefruit, raw, ½ medium, 3.3 ozs.	25	0	5
Grapefruit juice, unsweetened, 1 cup, 8 ozs.	48	0	22
Grapes, green, 1 cup, 3 ozs.	46 (av)	0	15
Kiwi, 1 medium, raw, peeled, 2½ ozs.	52 (av)	0	8
Lychee, canned and drained, 7	79	0	16
Mango, 1 small, 5 ozs.	55 (av)	0	19
Marmalade, 1 tablespoon	48	0	17
Orange, navel, 1 medium, 4 ozs.	44 (av)	0	10
Orange juice, 1 cup, 8 ozs.	46	0	26
Papaya, ½ medium, 5 ozs.	58 (av)	0	14
Peach, fresh, 1 medium, 3 ozs.	30	0	7
canned, natural juice, ½ cup, 4 ozs.	30	0	14
canned, light syrup, ½ cup, 4 ozs.	52	0	18
canned, heavy syrup, ½ cup, 4 ozs.	58	0	26
Pear, fresh, 1 medium, 5 ozs.	38 (av)	0	21
canned in pear juice, ½ cup, 4 ozs.	44	0	13
Pineapple, fresh, 2 slices, 4 ozs.	66	0	10
Pineapple juice, unsweetened, canned, 8 ozs.	46	0	34
Plums, 1 medium, 2 ozs.	39 (av)	0	7
Prunes, pitted, 6	29	0	25
Raisins, ¼ cup, 1 oz.	64	0	28
Strawberry jam, 1 tablespoon	51	0	18
Watermelon, 1 cup, 5 ozs.	72	0	8
Gatorade™ sports drink, 1 cup, 8 ozs.	78	0	14
Glucose powder, 2½ tablets	102	0	10
Gluten-free bread, 1 slice, 1 oz.	90	1	18
Glutinous rice, white, steamed, 1 cup	98	0	37
Gnocchi, cooked, 1 cup, 5 ozs.	68	3	71
Golden Grahams™, General Mills, ¾ cup, 1.6 ozs.	71	1	25
Graham crackers, 4 squares, 1 oz.	74	3	22
Granola Bars™, Quaker Chewy, 1 oz.	61	2	23
Grapefruit, raw, ½ medium, 3.3 ozs.	25	0	5
Grapefruit juice unsweetened, 1 cup, 8 ozs.	48	0	22
Grapenuts™, Post, breakfast cereal, ½ cup, 1 oz.	71	1	47
Grapenuts Flakes™, Post, breakfast cereal, ¾ cup, 1 oz.	80	1	24

THE GLUCOSE REVOLUTION POCKET GUIDE

Food	Glycemic Index	Fat (g per svg.)	CHO (g per svg.)
Grapes, green, 1 cup, 3.3 ozs.	46 (av)	0	15
Green pea soup, canned, ready to serve, 1 cup, 9 ozs.	66	3	27
Hamburger bun, 1 prepacked bun, 1½ ozs.	61	2	22
Honey, 1 tablespoon	58	0	16
Ice cream, 10% fat, vanilla, ½ cup, 2.2 ozs.	61 (av)	7	16
Ice milk, vanilla, ½ cup, 2.2 ozs.	50	3	15
Isostar, 1 cup, 8 ozs.	70	0	18
Jasmine, white, long grain, steamed, 1 cup	109	0	39
Jelly beans, 10 large, 1 oz.	80	0	26
Just Right™, breakfast cereal, ¾ cup	60	1	36
Kaiser rolls, 1 roll, 2 ozs.	73	2	34
Kavli™ All Natural Whole Grain Crispbread, 4 wafers, 1 oz.	71	1	16
Kidney beans, red, boiled, ½ cup, 3 ozs.	27 (av)	0	20
Kidney beans, red, canned and drained, ½ cup, 4.3 ozs.	52	0	19
Kiwi, 1 medium, raw, peeled, 2½ ozs.	52 (av)	0	8
Kudos Granola Bars™ (whole grain), 1 bar, 1 oz.	62	5	20
Lactose, pure, 7/10 oz.	46 (av)	0	10
Lentil soup, Unico, canned, 1 cup, 8 ozs.	44	1	24
Lentils, green and brown, boiled, ½ cup, 3 ozs.	30 (av)	0	16
Lentils, red, boiled, 1.4 cup, 4 ozs.	26 (av)	0	27
Life™, Quaker, breakfast cereal, ¾ cup, 1 oz.	66	1	25
Life Savers™, roll candy, 6 pieces, peppermint	70	0	10
Light deli (American) rye bread, 1 slice, 1 oz.	68	1	16
Lima beans, baby, frozen, ½ cup, 3 ozs.	32	0	17
Linguine pasta, thick, cooked, 1 cup, 6 ozs.	46 (av)	1	56
Linguine pasta, thin, cooked, 1 cup, 6 ozs.	55 (av)	1	56
Lychee, canned and drained, 7	79	0	16
M&M's Chocolate Candies Peanut™, 1.7 oz. package	33	13	30
Macaroni and Cheese Dinner™, Kraft packaged, cooked, 1 cup, 7 ozs.	64	17	48
Macaroni, cooked, 1 cup, 6 ozs.	45	1	42
Maltose (maltodextrin), pure, 2½ teaspoons	105	0	10
Mango, 1 small, 5 ozs.	55 (av)	0	19
Marmalade, 1 tablespoon	48	0	17
Mars Almond Bar™, 1.8 ozs.	65	12	31
Mars Bar™, 1 bar	65	11	41
Melba toast, 6 pieces, 1 oz.	70	1	23

CHILDREN WITH TYPE 1 DIABETES 137

Food	Glycemic Index	Fat (g per svg.)	CHO (g per svg.)
Milk, whole, 1 cup, 8 ozs.	27 (av)	9	11
skim, 1 cup, 8 ozs.	32	0	12
chocolate flavored, 1%, 1 cup, 8 ozs.	34	3	26
Milk Arrowroot, 3 cookies, ½ oz.	63	2	9
Millet, cooked, ½ cup, 4 ozs.	71	1	28
Mini Wheats (whole wheat), breakfast cereal, 1 cup	58	0	21
Muesli, breakfast cereal, toasted, ⅔ cup, 2 ozs.	43	3	41
Muesli, non-toasted, ⅔ cup, 1½ ozs.	56	3	28
Multi-Bran Chex™, General Mills, 1 cup, 2. ozs.	58	1.5	49
Muffins			
Apple cinnamon, from mix, 1 muffin, 2 ozs.	44	8	33
Apricot and honey, low fat, from mix, 1 muffin	60	4	27
Banana, oat and honey, low fat, from mix, 1 muffin, small	65	4	28
Blueberry, 1 muffin, 2 ozs.	59	4	27
Bran, 1 muffin	60	8	34
Chocolate butterscotch, low fat, from mix, 1 muffin	53	4	28
Oat and raisin, low fat, from mix, 1 muffin	54	3	28
Oat bran, 1 muffin, 2 ozs.	60	4	28
Mung beans, boiled, ½ cup, 3½ ozs.	38	1	18
Mung bean noodles, 1 cup	39	0	35
Natural Ovens 100% Whole Grain bread, 1 slice, 1.2 ozs.	51	0	17
Natural Ovens Hunger Filler bread, 1 slice, 1.2 ozs.	59	0	16
Natural Ovens Natural Wheat bread, 1 slice, 1.2 ozs.	59	0	16
Natural Ovens Happiness bread, 1 slice, 1.1 ozs.	63	0	15
Navy beans, boiled, ½ cup, 3 ozs.	38 (av)	0	19
Noodles, mung bean, 1 cup	39	0	35
Nutella™ (spread), 2 tablespoons	33	9	19
Nutri-grain™ breakfast cereal, 1 cup	66	0	20
Oat and raisin muffin, low fat from mix, 1 muffin	54	3	28
Oat bran, 1 tablespoon	55	1	7
Oat bran™, Quaker Oats, breakfast cereal, ¾ cup, 1 oz.	50	1	23
Oat bran, 1 muffin, 2 ozs.	60	4	28
Oatmeal (made with water), old fashioned, cooked, ½ cup, 4 ozs.	49	1	12
Oatmeal cookie, 1, ⅖ oz.	55	3	12
Oats, 1-minute, Quaker Oats, 1 cup, cooked	66	2	25
Orange, navel, 1 medium, 4 ozs.	44 (av)	0	10

THE GLUCOSE REVOLUTION POCKET GUIDE

Food	Glycemic Index	Fat (g per svg.)	CHO (g per svg.)
Orange syrup, diluted, 1 cup	66	0	20
Orange juice, 1 cup, 8 ozs.	46	0	26
Papaya, ½ medium, 5 ozs.	58 (av)	0	14
Parsnips, boiled, ½ cup, 2½ ozs.	97	0	15
Pasta			
Capellini, cooked, 1 cup, 6 ozs.	45	1	53
Fettuccine, cooked, 1 cup, 6 ozs.	32	1	57
Gnocchi, cooked, 1 cup, 5 ozs.	68	3	71
Linguine thick, cooked, 1 cup, 6 ozs.	46 (av)	1	56
Linguine thin, cooked, 1 cup, 6 ozs.	55 (av)	1	56
Macaroni, cooked, 1 cup, 5 ozs.	45	1	42
Macaroni & Cheese Dinner™, Kraft, packaged, cooked, 1 cup, 7 ozs.	64	17	48
Ravioli, meat-filled, cooked, 4 large	39	6	41
Spaghetti, white, cooked, 1 cup, 6 ozs.	41 (av)	1	42
Spaghetti, whole wheat, cooked, 1 cup, 6 ozs.	37 (av)	1	48
Spirali, durum, cooked, 1 cup, 6 ozs.	43	1	56
Star Pastina, cooked, 1 cup, 6 ozs.	38	1	56
Tortellini, cheese, cooked, 8 ozs.	50	7	28
Vermicelli, cooked, 1 cup, 6 ozs.	35	0	42
Pastry, flaky, ⅛ of double crust, 2 ozs.	59	15	24
Pea soup, split with ham, canned, 1 cup, 5½ ozs.	66	3	25
Peach, fresh, 1 medium, 3 ozs.	30	0	7
canned, heavy syrup, ½ cup, 4 ozs.	58	0	26
canned, light syrup, ½ cup, 4 ozs.	52	0	18
canned, natural juice, ½ cup, 4 ozs.	30	0	14
Peanuts, roasted, salted, ½ cup, 1.1 oz. bag	15 (av)	38	7
Pear, fresh, 1 medium, 5 ozs.	38 (av)	0	21
canned in pear juice, ½ cup, 4 ozs.	44	0	13
Peas, green, fresh, frozen, boiled, ½ cup, 2.7 ozs.	48 (av)	0	10
Peas dried, boiled, ½ cup, 2 ozs.	22	0	12
Pineapple, fresh, 2 slices, 4 ozs.	66	0	10
Pineapple juice, unsweetened, canned, 8 ozs.	46	0	34
Pinto beans, canned, ½ cup, 4 ozs.	45	1	18
Pinto beans, soaked, boiled, ½ cup, 3 ozs.	39	0	22
Pita bread, whole wheat, 6½ inch loaf, 2 ozs.	57	2	35

CHILDREN WITH TYPE 1 DIABETES

Food	Glycemic Index	Fat (g per svg.)	CHO (g per svg.)
Pizza, cheese and tomato, 2 slices, 8 ozs.	60	22	56
Pizza, Super Supreme, Pizza Hut, pan, 2 slices	36	31	72
Pizza, Super Supreme, Pizza Hut, thin and crispy, 2 slices	30	27	50
Plums, 1 medium, 2 ozs.	39 (av)	0	7
Popcorn, light, microwave, 1¾ oz. snack size	55	8	30
Pop Tarts™, double chocolate, 1 tart	70	5	36
Potatoes			
Desirée, peeled, boiled, 1 medium, 4 ozs.	101	0	13
French fries, large, 4.3 ozs.	75	26	49
instant mashed potatoes, Carnation Foods™, ½ cup, 3½ ozs.	86	2	14
new, unpeeled, boiled, 4 medium, 6 ozs.	78 (av)	0	25
new, canned, drained, 5 small, 6 ozs.	61	0	26
red-skinned, peeled, boiled, 1 medium, 4 ozs.	88 (av)	0	15
red-skinned, baked in oven (no fat), 1 medium, 4 ozs.	93 (av)	0	15
red-skinned, mashed, ½ cup, 4 ozs.	91 (av)	0	16
red-skinned, microwaved, 1 medium, 4 ozs.	79	0	15
sweet potato, peeled, boiled, mashed, ½ cup 3 ozs.	54 (av)	0	20
white-skinned, peeled, boiled, 1 medium, 4 ozs.	63 (av)	0	24
white-skinned, with skin, baked in oven (no fat), 1 medium, 4 ozs.	85 (av)	0	30
white-skinned, mashed, ½ cup, 4 ozs.	70 (av)	0	20
white-skinned, with skin, microwaved, 1 medium, 4 ozs.	82	0	29
Sebago, peeled, boiled, 1 medium, 4 ozs.	87	0	13
Potato chips, plain, 14 pieces, 1 oz.	54 (av)	10	15
Pound cake, 1 slice, homemade, 3 ozs.	54	15	42
Power Bar™, Performance, Chocolate, 1 bar	58	2	45
Premium saltine crackers, 8 crackers, 1 oz.	74	3	17
Pretzels, 1 oz.	83	1	22
Prunes, pitted, 6	29	0	25
Puffed Wheat™, Quaker, breakfast cereal, 2 cups, 1 oz.	80	0	22
Pumpernickel bread, whole grain, 2 slices	51	2	32
Pumpkin, peeled, boiled, mashed, ½ cup, 4 ozs.	75	0	6
Raisins, ¼ cup, 1 oz.	64	0	28
Raisin Bran™, Kellogg's, breakfast cereal, ¾ cup, 1.3 ozs.	73	0	32
Ravioli, meat-filled, cooked, 4 large	39	6	41

THE GLUCOSE REVOLUTION POCKET GUIDE

Food	Glycemic Index	Fat (g per svg.)	CHO (g per svg.)
Rice			
Arborio risotto rice, white, boiled, ⅔ cup	69	0	35
Basmati, white, boiled, 1 cup, 7 ozs.	58	0	50
Brown, 1 cup, 6 ozs.	55 (av)	0	37
Converted™, Uncle Ben's, 1 cup, 6 ozs.	44	0	38
Glutinous, white, steamed, 1 cup	98	0	37
Instant, cooked, 1 cup, 6 ozs.	87	0	38
Jasmine, white, long grain, steamed, 1 cup	109	0	39
Long grain, white, 1 cup, 6 ozs.	56 (av)	0	42
Parboiled, extruded, 1 cup, 6 ozs.	48	0	38
Rice bran, extruded, 1 tablespoon	19	2	3
Rice cakes, plain, 3 cakes, 1 oz.	82	1	23
Short grain, white, 1 cup, 6 ozs.	72	0	42
Rice Chex™, General Mills, breakfast cereal, 1¼ cups, 1 oz.	89	0	27
Rice Krispies™, Kellogg's, breakfast cereal, 1¼ cups, 1 oz.	82	0	26
Rice vermicelli, cooked, 6 ozs.	58	0	48
Roll (bread), Kaiser, 1 roll, 2 ozs.	73	2	39
Roll-ups™, 1 fruit leather	99	1	13
Romano (cranberry) beans, boiled, ½ cup, 3 ozs.	46	0	21
Rutabaga, peeled, boiled, ½ cup, 2.6 ozs.	72	0	3
Rye bread, 1 slice, 1 oz.	65	1	15
Ryvita™ Tasty Dark Rye Whole Grain Crisp Bread, 2 slices, ⅔ oz.	69	1	16
Semolina, cooked, 1 cup, 6 ozs.	55	0	17
Shortbread, 4 small cookies, 1 oz.	64	7	19
Shredded Wheat™, Post, breakfast cereal, 1 oz.	83	1	23
Shredded wheat, 1 biscuit, ⅘ oz.	62	0	19
Shredded wheat, spoonsize, 1 cup, 1.2 ozs.	58	0	27
Skittles Original Fruit Bite Size Candies™, 2.3 oz. pk.	70	3	59
Smacks™, Kellogg's, breakfast cereal, ¾ cup, 1 oz.	56	1	27
Snickers™, 2.2 oz. bar	41	15	36
Social Tea™ biscuits, Nabisco, 4 cookies, ⅔ oz.	55	3	13
Soft drink, Coca-Cola™, 1 can, 12 ozs.	63	0	39
Soft drink, Fanta™, 1 can, 12 ozs.	68	0	47
Soups			
Black bean soup, ½ cup, 4½ ozs.	64	2	19
Green pea soup, canned, ready to serve, 1 cup, 9 ozs.	66	3	27

CHILDREN WITH TYPE 1 DIABETES

Food	Glycemic Index	Fat (g per svg.)	CHO (g per svg.)
Lentil soup, Unico, canned, 1 cup, 8 ozs.	44	1	24
Pea soup, split with ham, 1 cup, 5½ ozs.	66	3	25
Tomato soup, canned, 1 cup, 9 ozs.	38	4	33
Sourdough bread, 1 slice, 1½ ozs.	52	1	20
Rye bread, Arnold's, 1 slice, 1½ ozs.	57	1	21
Soy beans, boiled, ½ cup, 3 ozs.	18 (av)	7	10
Soy milk, 1 cup, 8 ozs.	31	7	14
Spaghetti, white, cooked, 1 cup	41 (av)	1	42
Spaghetti, whole wheat, cooked, 1 cup, 5 ozs.	37 (av)	1	48
Special K™, Kellogg's, breakfast cereal, 1 cup, 1 oz.	54	0	22
Spirali, durum, cooked, 1 cup, 6 ozs.	43	1	56
Split pea soup, 8 ozs.	60	4	38
Split peas, yellow, boiled, ½ cup, 3½ ozs.	32	0	29
Sponge cake plain, 1 slice, 3½ ozs.	46	4	32
Sports drinks			
Gatorade™ 1 cup, 8 ozs.	78	0	14
Isostar, 1 cup, 8 ozs.	70	0	18
Sportsplus, 1 cup, 8 ozs.	74	0	17
Power Bar™, Performance Chocolate Bar, 1 bar	58	3	45
Stoned wheat thins, 3 crackers, ⅘ oz.	67	2	15
Strawberry Nestle Quik™ (made with water), 3 teaspoons	64	0	14
Strawberry jam, 1 tablespoon	51	0	18
Sucrose, 1 teaspoon	65 (av)	0	4
Super Supreme pizza, Pizza Hut, pan, 2 slices	36	31	72
Super Supreme pizza, Pizza Hut, thin and crispy, 2 slices	30	27	50
Syrup, fruit flavored, diluted, 1 cup	66	0	20
Sweet potato, peeled, boiled, mashed, ½ cup 3 ozs.	54 (av)	0	20
Taco shells, 2 shells, 1 oz.	68	5	17
Tapioca pudding, boiled with whole milk, 1 cup, 10 ozs.	81	13	51
Taro, peeled, boiled, ½ cup, 2 ozs.	54	0	23
Team Flakes™, Nabisco, breakfast cereal, ¾ cup, 1 oz.	82	0	25
Tofu frozen dessert, nondairy, low fat, 2 ozs.	115	1	21
Tomato soup, canned, 1 cup, 9 ozs.	38	4	33
Tortellini, cheese, cooked, 8 ozs.	50	7	28
Total™, General Mills, breakfast cereal, ¾ cup, 1 oz.	76	1	24
Twix Chocolate Caramel Cookie™, 2, 2 ozs.	44	14	37
Vanilla wafers, 7 cookies, 1 oz.	77	4	21

Food	Glycemic Index	Fat (g per svg.)	CHO (g per svg.)
Vermicelli, cooked, 1 cup, 6 ozs.	35	0	42
Vitasoy™ Soy milk, creamy original, 1 cup, 8 ozs.	31	7	14
Waffles, plain, frozen, 4 inch square, 1 oz.	76	3	13
Water crackers, 3 king size crackers, ⅘ oz.	78	2	18
Watermelon, 1 cup, 5 ozs.	72	0	8
Weetabix™ breakfast cereal, 2 biscuits, 1.2 ozs.	75	1	28
White bread, 1 slice, 1 oz.	70 (av)	1	12
Whole wheat bread, 1 slice, 1 oz.	69 (av)	1	13
Yam, boiled, 3 oz.	51	0	24
Yogurt			
nonfat, fruit flavored, with sugar, 8 ozs.	33	0	30
nonfat, plain, artificial sweetener, 8 ozs.	14	0	17
nonfat, fruit flavored, artificial sweetener, 8 ozs.	14	0	17

FOR MORE INFORMATION

*I*f you'd like to know the glycemic index of more foods, write to the food manufacturer and encourage them to contact:

SYDNEY UNIVERSITY GLYCEMIC INDEX RESEARCH SERVICE (SUGIRS)

Dr. Jennie Brand-Miller
Department of Biochemistry
University of Sydney
NSW 2006 Australia
Fax: (61) (2) 9351-6022
E-mail: j.brandmiller@staff.usyd.edu.au
Website:
www.biochem.usyd.edu.au/~jennie/GI/glycemic
_index.html

REGISTERED DIETITIANS

Registered Dietitians (RDs) are nutrition experts who provide nutritional assessment and guidance and support. Check for the initials "RD" after the name to identify qualified dietitians who provide the highest standard of care to their clients. Glycemic index is part of their training so all dietitians should be able to help in applying the principles in this guide, but some dietitians do specialize in certain areas. If you want more detailed advice on glycemic index just ask the dietitian whether this is a specialty when you make your appointment.

Dietitians work in hospitals and often run their own private practices, as well. For a list of dietitians in your area, contact the American Dietetic Association (ADA)'s Consumer Nutrition Hotline (1-800-366-1655) or visit ADAs home page at the address below. You can also check the Yellow Pages under "Dietitians."

The American Dietetic Association
216 West Jackson Boulevard
Chicago, IL 60606
Phone: 1-800-877-1600
Fax: 1-312-899-1979
Website: http://www.eatright.org/

PRIMARY CARE PHYSICIANS

It's always a good idea to discuss any health problems or concerns with your primary care physician.

WEIGHT LOSS ORGANIZATIONS

To help your child lose weight, check the Yellow Pages under "Weight Control Services." Be aware, however, that not all weight loss organizations are reputable. Check with your physician to make sure the group you would like your child to join can help her lose weight safely.

CHILDREN WITH TYPE 1 DIABETES

DIABETES ORGANIZATIONS

Extra weight can often make a diabetic condition worse. For more information about living with and controlling diabetes, contact the following:

The American Diabetes Association
1660 Duke Street
Alexandria, VA 22314
Phone: 1-800-ADA-DISC (1-800-232-3472)
Website: http://www.diabetes.org/
Canadian Diabetes Association National Office
15 Toronto Street Suite #800
Toronto, ON M5C 2E3
Phone: 1-416-363-3373
1-800-BANTING (1-800-226-8464)
Website: http://www.diabetes.ca/

NATURAL OVENS ORDERING INFORMATION

Natural Ovens of Manitowoc
4300 County Trunk CR
P.O. Box 730
Manitowoc WI 54221-073
Telephone: 1-800-772-0730
Fax: 1-920-758-2594
Website: http://www.naturalovens.com/

ABOUT THE AUTHORS

Heather Gilbertson, B. Sc., Grad. Dip. Diet., Grad. Cert. Diab. Ed., APD, an accredited practicing dietitian and diabetes educator, has extensive experience in diabetes management in children and adolescents and has researched the effect of low glycemic index and measured carbohydrate diets in children with diabetes. She currently works at the Women's and Children's Health Care Network, Royal Children's Hospital Campus, Melbourne, and conducts a private practice in the Macedon Ranges, Victoria, Australia.

Jennie Brand-Miller, Ph.D., Associate Professor of Human Nutrition in the Human Nutrition Unit, Department of Biochemistry, University of Sydney, Australia, is a world authority on the glycemic index of foods. She received her B.Sc. (1975) and Ph.D. (1979) degrees from the Department of Food Science and Technology at the University of New South Wales, Australia. She is the editor of the *Proceedings of the Nutrition Society of Australia* and a member of the Scientific Consultative Committee of the Australian Nutrition Foundation. She has written more than 200 research papers, including 60 on the glycemic index of foods. A co-author of *The Glucose Revolution* and all the titles in The Glucose Revolution Pocket Guide series, she lives in Sydney, Australia. Her most recent book is *The Glucose Revolution Life Plan*.

Kaye Foster-Powell, B. Sc., M.Nutr. & Diet, is an accredited practicing dietitian-nutritionist. A graduate of the University of Sydney (B.Sc., 1987; Master of Nutrition and Dietetics, 1994), she has extensive experience in diabetes management and has completed lengthy research on practical applications of the glycemic index. She is the senior dietitian at Wentworth Area Diabetes Service and conducts a private practice in the Blue Mountains, New South Wales. Her most recent book is *The Glucose Revolution Life Plan*.

Thomas M.S. Wolever, M.D., Ph.D., another of the world's leading researchers of the glycemic index, is Professor in the Department of Nutritional Sciences, University of Toronto, and a member of the Division of Endocrinology and Metabolism, St. Michael's Hospital, Toronto. He is a graduate of Oxford University (B.A., M.A., M.B., B. Ch., M.Sc., and D.M.) in the United Kingdom. He received his Ph.D. at the University of Toronto. His research since 1980 has focused on the glycemic index of foods and the prevention of type 2 diabetes. A co-author of *The Glucose Revolution* and all the titles in The Glucose Revolution Pocket Guide series, he lives in Toronto, Canada.

Johanna Burani, M.S., R.D., C.D.E., is a registered dietitian and certified diabetes educator with more than 11 years experience in nutritional counseling. She specializes in designing individual meal plans based on low G.I. food choices. The adapter of *The Glucose Revolution* and the co-adapter, with Linda Rao, of all the titles in The Glucose Revolution Pocket Guide series, she is the author of seven books and professional manuals, and lives in Mendham,

New Jersey. Her most recent book is *The Glucose Revolution Life Plan*.

Linda Rao, M.Ed., a freelance writer and editor, has been writing and researching health topics for the past 12 years. Her work has appeared in several national publications, including *Prevention*, *Cooking Light*, and *USA Today*. She serves as a contributing editor for *Prevention* magazine and is the co-adapter, with Johanna Burani, of all the titles in The Glucose Revolution Pocket Guide series. She lives in Allentown, Pennsylvania.

ACKNOWLEDGMENTS

We would like to acknowledge the extraordinary efforts of Johanna Burani and Linda Rao, who adapted this book—and the other books in The Glucose Revolution Pocket Guide series—for North American readers. Together they have worked to ensure that every piece of information is accurate and appropriate for readers in the U.S. and Canada.

For more information about *The Glucose Revolution*, *The Glucose Revolution Life Plan*, and *The Glucose Revolution Pocket Guides*, visit **www.glucoserevolution.com**

The Glucose Revolution begins here...

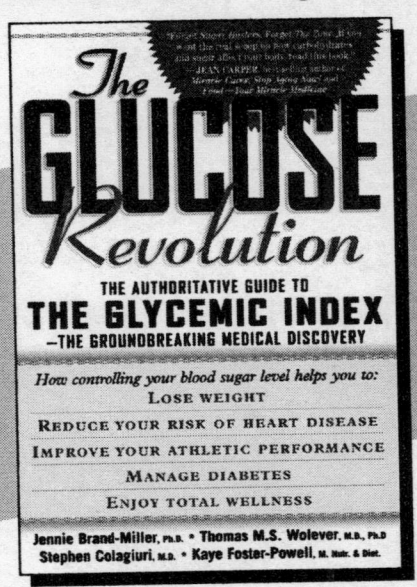

THE GLUCOSE REVOLUTION
THE AUTHORITATIVE GUIDE TO THE GLYCEMIC INDEX— THE GROUNDBREAKING MEDICAL DISCOVERY

NATIONAL BESTSELLER!

"Forget *Sugar Busters*. Forget *The Zone*. If you want the real scoop on how carbohydrates and sugar affect your body, read this book by the world's leading researchers on the subject. It's the authoritative, last word on choosing foods to control your blood sugar."

—JEAN CARPER, best-selling author of *Miracle Brain, Miracle Cures, Stop Aging Now!* and *Food—Your Miracle Medicine*

ISBN 1-56924-660-2 • $14.95

. . . and continues with these other *Glucose Revolution Pocket Guides*

The Glucose Revolution Pocket Guide to
LOSING WEIGHT

Eat yourself slim with low glycemic index foods

Not all foods are created equal when it comes to losing weight. The latest medical research shows that carbohydrates with a low glycemic index have special advantages because they fill you up and keep you satisfied longer. This pocket guide will help you eat yourself slim with low glycemic index foods and show you how low glycemic index foods make sustained weight loss possible. This guide also includes a 7-day low glycemic index plan for losing weight, G.I. success stories, and the glycemic index and fat and carbohydrate content of more than 300 foods and drinks.

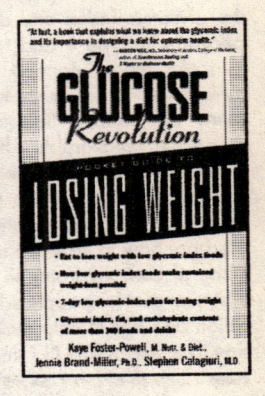

ISBN 1-56924-677-7 • $4.95

The Glucose Revolution Pocket Guide to
SPORTS NUTRITION

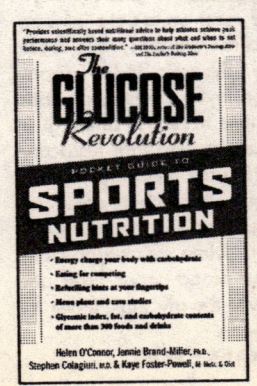

Eat to compete better than ever before.

Serious athletes and weekend warriors can gain a winning edge by manipulating the glycemic index of their diets. Now this at-a-glance guide shows how to use the glycemic index to boost athletic performance, enhance stamina, and prevent fatigue. Subjects covered include energy charging with carbohydrates, eating for competing, refueling hints, menu plans and case studies, and the glycemic index, fat and carbohydrate content of more than 300 foods and drinks.

ISBN 1-56924-676-9 • $4.95

The Glucose Revolution Pocket Guide to
DIABETES

Help control your diabetes with low glycemic index foods

Based on the most up-to-date information about carbohydrates, this basic guide to the glycemic index and diabetes allows people with type 1 and type 2 diabetes to make more informed choices about their diets. Topics covered include why many traditionally "taboo" foods don't cause the unfavorable effects on blood sugar levels they were believed to have, and why diets based on low G.I. foods improve blood sugar control. Also covered are how to include more of the right kinds of carbohydrates in your diet, the optimum diet for people with diabetes, practical hints for meal preparation and tips to help make the glycemic index work throughout the day, a week of low G.I. menus, G.I. success stories, and more.

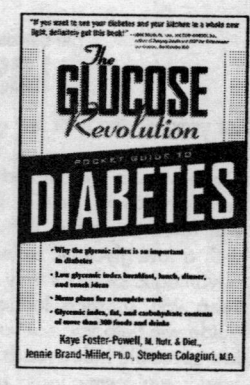

ISBN 1-56924-675-0 • $4.95

The Glucose Revolution Pocket Guide to
SUGAR AND ENERGY

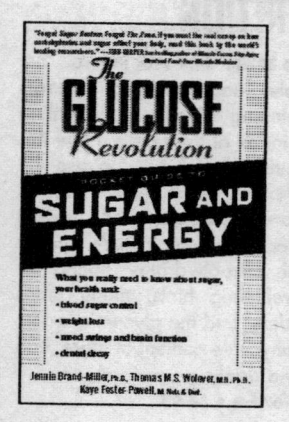

Sugar's off the black list—find out why

Based on the most up-to-date information about carbohydrates, this basic guide to the glycemic index dispels many common myths about sugar and why it's high time to get rid of the guilt. With evidence showing that restricting refined sugar in your diet may do more harm than good, the authors show you how to intelligently give in to your sugar cravings and regulate your sugar intake to control your blood sugar level and lose weight, with the glycemic index for nearly 150 foods.

ISBN 1-56924-641-6 • $4.95

The Glucose Revolution Pocket Guide to
THE TOP 100 LOW GLYCEMIC FOODS

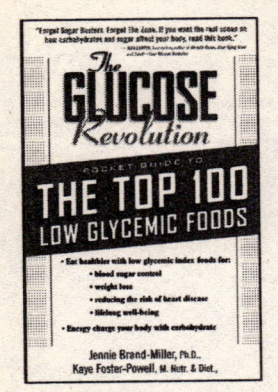

ISBN 1-56924-678-5 • $4.95

The best of the best in low glycemic index foods

The slow digestion and gradual rise and fall in blood sugar levels after a food with a low glycemic index has benefits for many people. Today we know the glycemic index of hundreds of different generic and name-brand foods, which have been tested following a standardized method. Now *The Top 100 Low Glycemic Foods* makes it easy to enjoy those slowly digested carbohydrates every day for better blood sugar control, weight loss, a healthy heart, and peak athletic performance.

The Glucose Revolution Pocket Guide to
THE GLYCEMIC INDEX AND HEALTHY KIDS

Give Your Child the Gift of Healthy Eating Habits

Getting children to eat and enjoy healthy foods is one of the challenges every parent faces daily. Now, the world's leading experts on the glycemic index (G.I.) explain how to improve and maintain your children's overall nutrition and health through the G.I. Topics covered include strategies for meeting kids' dietary needs without conflict and the specific nutrition needs for children of all ages. Complete with simple meal plans and recipes that will help maintain your child's energy levels steady all day, *The Glucose Revolution Pocket Guide to the Glycemic Index and Healthy Kids* will help you to foster lifelong healthy eating habits in your children.

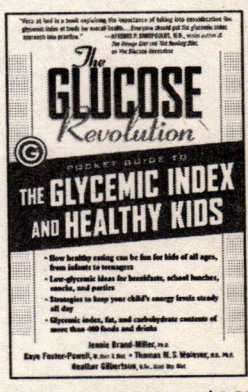

ISBN 1-56924-588-6 • $4.95

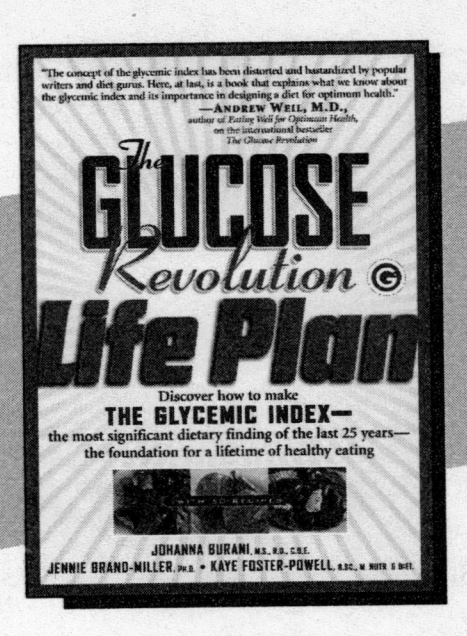

THE GLUCOSE REVOLUTION LIFE PLAN

DISCOVER HOW TO MAKE THE GLYCEMIC INDEX—THE MOST SIGNIFICANT DIETARY FINDING OF THE LAST 25 YEARS—THE FOUNDATION FOR A LIFETIME OF HEALTHY EATING

Both an introduction to the benefits of low-G.I. foods and an essential source for those already familiar with the concept, *The Glucose Revolution Life Plan* presents the glycemic index within the context of today's full nutrition picture. With the glycemic index as its starting point, it gives readers clear guidelines for choosing the diet that is right for them. With the most authoritative, up-to-date and complete table of G.I. values published anywhere, *The Glucose Revolution Life Plan* makes the glycemic index accessible and useful to more readers than ever before.

ISBN 1-56924-609-2 • $18.95